MORALITY IN MEDICINE

An Introduction to Medical Ethics

MORALITY IN MEDICINE

An Introduction to Medical Ethics

RICHARD WARNER
UNIVERSITY OF PENNSYLVANIA

Printed and bound in the United States of America

Library of Congress Cataloging in Publication Data

Warner, Richard, 1946–
Morality in medicine.

Includes index.
1. Medical ethics. 2. Informed consent (Medical law)
I. Title.
R724.W34   174'.2   79-23049
ISBN 0-88284-103-3

TO MY PARENTS

ACKNOWLEDGEMENTS

There are numerous friends and colleagues with whom
I have discussed the issues and problems examined in this
book; however, there are four people who should be
singled out. Nancy Hanke, M.D. gave me very accurate
and helpful comments and criticisms at all stages
of the manuscript's preparation. She also encouraged
and tolerated me throughout the writing of the
book. My father, Judge Verne Warner, also read the
entire manuscript and gave me invaluable advice
on legal points. The entire manuscript was also read
by Suzy Breyer, R.N., and I should thank her for
timely criticism and encouragement. Finally, I should
thank Joe Volpe for many discussions which
were helpful in writing the Introduction.

In addition, I should thank three restaurants. The
two in which the book was written for their coffee and
hospitality—Kelly and Cohen's, and Fiesta Pizza.
And one in which the book was not written, La Terrasse.

I also owe thanks to Andrea MacFarland, Diane
Stillwell, Lore Silverberg and Duane Williams for
excellent and patient typing and retyping.

CONTENTS

PREFACE

Moral problems arise in the practice of medicine, and consent is one central concept which appears repeatedly in the analysis of these problems. A person has the right to give or withhold consent to medical treatment, and this right is a focal point where many separate moral issues intersect. Accordingly, Chapter 1 considers the right to consent. Why does it exist? And what does it imply? The issue of consent also plays a central role in the discussion of euthanasia (Chapter 2), abortion (Chapter 3), and the rights of mental patients (Chapter 4). The right to consent only recedes into the background in Chapter 5 where we discuss the right to health care and its implications. This right provides a convenient vantage point from which we can survey the social issues raised by health care. By focusing on the problems of social decision, Chapter 5 differs from the other chapters, which are concerned primarily with decisions which affect, and which are made by, a single individual or small group of individuals. So, the book ends with a transition from the individual to the social perspective.

While I think this book should be of interest to professional philosophers, it was not written primarily for them. The book was written for nonphilosophers, especially doctors, nurses, students, patients, and so on. However, it differs from many books aimed at nonphilosophers in paying a fair amount of attention to moral theory. My experience teaching practical ethics has convinced me that people want to see that things rest on a solid foundation. The book begins with an introduction which outlines its basic theoretical framework, and each chapter ends with a section on theoretical foundations. These sections discuss in more detail some central theoretical point or assumption made in the chapter. Those with a taste for theory will probably dislike having these discussions relegated to the end of the chapter. But people differ greatly in their tolerance for theoretical investigations, and the sections on theoretical foundations seemed a good compromise. It is worth remarking that the theoretical framework is built upon psychological facts about people. This explains the unusual number of quotes from Carl Jung which appear in the book. Jung had deep concern with morality and its connection to psychology, and his writings contain much that is valuable to the philosophical foundations of morality.

To write a book about moral problems, you must (or at least, you should) articulate your conception of how to live. I think this is worth doing since it is my conviction that a person should have a conscious conception of how to live. Of course, I do not expect you to agree completely with this conception of how to live. This is especially true because this is a book aimed at nonphilosophers. In such a book, ideas stand out starkly and clearly without all the trappings of professional philosophy. The book will serve its purpose if, where you disagree, you develop your own conception of what is morally right.

A final stylistic note. Philosophers often use the expression, "A if and only if B" to express the fact that A and B are equivalent. This "if and only if" is accurate but stylistically awkward. So, I have often used "provided that" as a replacement for it. This stylistic variation should cause no confusion.

Richard Warner
Philadelphia
January, 1980

MORALITY IN MEDICINE

An Introduction to Medical Ethics

Introduction

*... to live is, in itself, a value
judgment. To breathe is to judge.*

—Albert Camus, *The Rebel*

An individual life is a pattern of choices. The pattern is complex and unique, and the choices may be explicit or implicit, conscious or unconscious. Some of these choices will be moral ones; that is, choices which raise the question: What ought I to do? It is typical of moral choices that this question is difficult to answer, and it is also typical that the answer matters. Abortion is a good example. If a woman decides against abortion, it may mean having an unwanted child. Deciding in favor of abortion, on the other hand, means that a person who would have been will not be. What should the woman do? It is not easy to answer this question, and the consequences make the answer matter.

This introduction will provide a theoretical framework in which to consider moral questions. Without such a framework we would be unable to explain adequately the reasons for our answers; we would have merely one more collection of unsupported opinions about morality. What we need, and what we aim at here, is a well-reasoned approach to moral issues—an approach which explains and makes sense of the moral choices we face. In addition, unless we have a solid understanding of the reasons for our ethical views, it is doubtful that we will deal effectively and consistently with moral problems and issues. Lacking solid understanding, we might very well be too easily swayed from our views when confronted with a forceful opponent who argued against us or when faced with a distasteful moral problem which it would be easier to ignore. A sound theoretical understanding, on the other hand, provides a solid foundation on which we can build a sound and consistent practice.

1. Why be moral?

A good theoretical foundation must answer the question: Why be moral? What does this question mean? An example will help. Suppose you drive by an old man whose car is stalled on the road and who

1

obviously needs help changing a tire. The road is deserted, and it is unlikely that anyone else will be passing by for several hours at least. In fact, the old man could be stranded there all night. But suppose also that it interferes with your pursuit of your self-interest to stop and help. You could do so, but it would be inconvenient since you are already late for dinner at a friend's. Also, you know that if you just drive on, you will feel guilty—but only for a few moments. Can we give you a reason which would show that you should stop and help—even though it interferes with your pursuit of your self-interest?

We can see that the question. Why be moral? arises when there is a conflict between self-interest and the answer to the question: What ought I to do? You may think that what you *ought* to do is stop and help, even though you can see clearly that doing so interrupts the plans that serve your self-interest. Still, we may begin to wonder why we should do what it first seems we ought to do. Maybe we should just act in ways that serve our self-interest. *Can we really give a good reason for acting in a way that interrupts our pursuit of our self-interest?* This was the question I had in mind when I asked, Why be moral? What we want to see is whether there can be a good reason to resolve this conflict on the side of morality.

This point is well illustrated by the following example. In the 1960s and seventies during the Vietnam war, men over eighteen faced the draft, and many refused to be inducted into the armed services. Many refused even though they knew it was definitely *not* in their self-interest to do so; for, as they knew, refusal generally meant prison or exile. Those who refused often gave as one of their reasons their belief that it was immoral to participate in any way in the Vietnam war. Now, how could this belief provide them with such a strong reason to act against their self-interest? How could it give them a reason to abandon their families, friends, and careers and accept prison and exile? Here we are not concerned with the truth of the belief that a person ought not to have participated in the war in Vietnam; what we are concerned with is the claim that this belief gave certain people a strong reason to act against their self-interest.

Now, if we understand the question: Why be moral? as asking: Can we have a good reason to interrupt our pursuit of self-interest? it certainly looks like the answer must be a flat denial that there is a good reason to be moral when being moral would conflict with self-interest. At least, many people are convinced that all good reasons for action must be based on self-interest. Let us call this *the self-interest view of reasons.* It is the view that all good reasons we can have for our actions must be based on the fact that the action is in our self-interest. This view does not deny that people may act for reasons other than those of self-interest. For example, a man may sacrifice his life to save someone else, and he may have all sorts of reasons for doing so. But unless it was in his self-interest to sacrifice his life, he didn't have a *good* reason. And so, in the draft resisters' case, for example, there are only two possibilities. Either they did not have a good reason to refuse the draft or it was in their self-interest to refuse.

In general, when we ask: Can we give a good reason to interrupt our pursuit of self-interest? it certainly seems that the self-interest view of reasons must answer with a clear *no*. If all good reasons derive from self-interest considerations, how could we have a good reason to interrupt our pursuit of our self-interest?

Should we accept the self-interest view of reasons? Perhaps that view is wrong. But I think we can demonstrate that it isn't. Consider the questions: Why should I do that? and Why should I care about that? We have all been involved in discussions in which a person keeps asking these questions over and over no matter how many reasons we give him for doing what we think he should do. Now, if he really ought to do what we think he should, if what we think he should do is not just a mere reflection of our own personal prejudices, then we should be able to answer his questions. But he can legitimately continue to raise these questions until we can show him that it is in his *self-interest* to do what we think he should do. We can always be forced back to his point when we attempt to provide a good reason. This is what makes the self-interest view of reasons plausible.

So, we will accept the self-interest view of reasons. But how does this view affect morality? Is there no reason to be moral when morality conflicts with our pursuit of self-interest? Recall the tire-changing example. Should you drive on and leave the old man stranded if it interfered with your pursuit of self-interest to stop and help? To answer this question *yes* is to have a cold and brutal view of human existence, but it is the view we will have to accept unless we can find a good reason to be moral even when the demands of morality conflict with considerations of self-interest. But how can we possibly find such a reason if we accept the self-interest view of reasons?

The solution to this dilemma lies in seeing that, appearances to the contrary, *it really is in our self-interest to be moral.* The idea that it is goes back at least to Plato. One of its recent exponents is the psycho-analyst Carl Jung, who insists that

> morality is not a misconception invented by some vaunting Moses on Sinai, but something inherent in the laws of life. . . . The vital optimum is not to be found in crude egoism, for fundamentally man is so constituted that the pleasure he gives his neighbor is something

essential to him. Nor can the optimum be reached by an unbridled craving for individualistic supremacy, because the collective element in man is so powerful that his longing for fellowship would destroy all pleasure in naked egoism.[1]

The idea is simple: You will be happier if you are moral rather than immoral. But we have just seen that the demands of morality frequently conflict with the pursuit of self-interest. So, how can it possibly be true *for everyone* that he or she will be happier if moral? How can it possibly be in our self-interest to be moral?

The answers lie in a better understanding of morality and self-interest. In the remainder of this chapter we will sketch out the argument that it is in our self-interest to be moral. (A full and complete argument would require a book-length theoretical treatment of its own.) A brief sketch is essential for at least two reasons. First, a work on practical moral problems such as this should be built on a solid theoretical foundation and should make its theoretical framework clear. Second, the question: Why be moral? is itself of great practical relevance. People want to know how to deal with the moral choices they face, and this is the first question they need an answer to. The answer they give makes a clear difference in the way they conduct their lives.

2. What it means to be moral

We want to argue that it is in our self-interest to be moral. But we can hardly hope to show that it is in our self-interest to be moral until we know what morality is.

So, let's put aside the question: Why be moral? for the time being and turn to the prior question about *meaning:* What do we mean when we talk about "being moral?" We can answer this question by imagining a person who rejects all morality, a person who thinks morality is just a mistake, an illusion. Imagine this person as never concerned with the happiness of others unless he thinks it will make *him* happier to do something that will make someone else happy. He runs his life in such a way that he never gives up anything he wants in order to promote the happiness of others unless he thinks he can get even more of what he wants by doing so. His happiness always comes first; he does not care whether others suffer as long as he gets what he wants. He realizes other people will regard him as immoral, but he thinks they are wrong because he rejects their concepts of morality. Such a person is an *amoralist;* he stands outside all systems of morality, refusing to adopt any moral point of view.

Now, I doubt that anyone is really a complete amoralist. All of us are ready to give up getting what we want at least some of the time for at least some people. Parents may give up getting the new car they want in order to pay their children's tuition at college. Or, you may give up buying new clothes in order to buy a present for someone you like. And so on. We often do such things because it will make someone else happy. We don't worry about whether it will lead to our getting more of what *we* want; increasing our happiness is not our motive—or at least not our main motive. In general, all of us are ready—some of the time and for some people—to put another's happiness before our own. And, to the extent we are ready to do this, we are not amoralists. *For the difference between an amoralist and a moral person is a readiness to put another's happiness before his own.* As soon as we imagine the amoralist as having a readiness to put another's happiness before his own, he no longer counts as a complete amoralist.

So, what you need to make you count as moral is a concern for happiness in general—my happiness as well as yours. And this is the answer to the question about what it means to be moral. *A moral person is ready to some degree to try to increase, to maximize, happiness in general.* But to count as a moral, as opposed to an amoral person, you only have to be ready to maximize happiness in general sometimes for some people.

But why should I try to maximize happiness in general—even only sometimes, for some people? Why shouldn't I just pursue my own self-interest? Why shouldn't I be an amoralist? The answer is that you should pursue your own self-interest, but it is in your self-interest to be moral, to be ready (sometimes) to maximize happiness in general. This is why you have a good reason to be moral.

3. Why be moral? A sketch of an answer

Why is it in our self-interest to be moral—to be ready to maximize happiness in general, not just our own happiness? We will argue that it is in our self-interest to be moral *because we have a strong need to be moral.* How can we convince ourselves this is so? The French writer Albert Camus approaches this question by a consideration of suicide. He first asks: What reason is there to continue to live and experience? and this will be our starting point as well. A consideration of suicide brings out the essential connection between our personal happiness and happiness in general.

Why should we continue to live and experience? There is always an alternative—namely, suicide. Should we continue to live instead of committing suicide? Since suicide is always an alternative, this question can be raised about any life—even the most successful and comfortable—although we do not normally do so. Of course, there are situations in which the question arises naturally; for example, that of a ninety-two-year-old man who is rapidly dying of cancer and who is in chronic, unrelievable, and intolerable pain.

But our interest here is not in such extreme situations; rather, it is in ordinary daily life. We want to focus on those situations in which we have reasonable prospects of success, comfort, pleasure, and enjoyment. What reason do we have to live such a life? One possible answer is: "I have good reason to live my life because I want to be happy, and because I have reasonable prospects of satisfying that desire." This is the first answer many people will think of. What this answer does is give us a *personal* reason to continue to live since it holds out before us the prospect of our own personal future happiness. Now, if this were a satisfactory answer to the question: Why continue to live? there would be no connection between that question and the question: Why be moral? But it is not a satisfactory answer. When a person asks: Why should I continue to live? what he wants is a *nonpersonal* reason to live—a reason which is not of the form "because I can satisfy *my* desires, because I can achieve *my* happiness." It is the need for a nonpersonal answer that connects the two questions. It is not at all obvious that this is so, but the connection is there, and it is important that we see it if we want to see why we should be moral.

We can begin to understand the connection by seeing why we need a nonpersonal reason to live. There can be no doubt that we do need such a reason. It is the idea that there is no such reason which leads to the feeling that life is empty and meaningless—the mere pointless pursuit of one's own happiness. Indeed, literary as well as religious traditions show that people desire to see their lives as having a rationale beyond the mere satisfaction of their own desires. The effect of not finding such a rationale is well illustrated by this passage from Kierkegaard's *Either/Or:*

The sun shines into my room bright and beautiful, the window is open in the next room; on the street all is quiet, it is a Sunday afternoon. Outside the window, I clearly hear a lark pour forth its song in a neighbor's garden, where the pretty maiden lives. Far away in a distant street I hear a man crying shrimps. The air is so warm, and yet the whole town seems dead. Then I think of my youth and of my first love—when the longing of desire was strong. Now I long only for my first longing. What is youth? A dream. What is love? The substance of a dream.[2]

Without a nonpersonal reason for living, life begins to seem like an empty and pointless dream.[3] We have a strong psychological need for a nonpersonal reason to live. What we want to affirm is that the life we have a personal reason to live—the life in which each of us pursues his or her own happiness—is also worth living from a nonpersonal point of view. We do not want to find reasons to continue to live simply in the fact that we can achieve our own happiness. Rather, what we want to affirm is that happiness in general is worth pursuing and should be maximized. Then, each of us would have a nonpersonal reason to live. Your reason for living would be "Because my happiness, and the happiness of others which I promote, will contribute to the sum total of happiness in general." This is *not* a personal reason of the form "because I can satisfy *my* desires."

To sum up: *We are claiming that we have a strong psychological need to affirm that we should maximize happiness in general.* In other words, we need to affirm that we should be moral. We have this need because we have the need for a nonpersonal reason to live.[4]

But what *reason* is there to affirm this? Our discussion has revealed a need to be moral, but how has it revealed a reason? Indeed, you may react to this whole discussion of morality by thinking we have made no progress at all. This is a natural reaction since it is natural to look for a foundation for morality outside people's needs; for example, people often look for a religious foundation which derives morality from the will of God. But this natural reaction is a bad reaction for two reasons. First, it is doubtful that there is a foundation for morality outside people's needs. Second, looking for a foundation outside people's needs makes us overlook the fact that our needs do give us an adequate foundation for morality. We need to affirm that we should be moral, *and that need itself gives us a good reason to affirm that we should.*

This is a crucial point, and it needs careful explanation. By affirming that we should be moral, I mean adopting as a rule of conduct the principle that happiness in general should be maximized. This does not mean just giving lip service to this rule; rather, it means being committed to trying to maximize happiness in general. It means actually living a moral life—not just saying that you should. Now, the essential point is that *this sort of commitment to the moral life satisfies—to some extent at least—the need for a nonpersonal reason to live.* This, I suggest, is a psychological fact.

In brief, we have a strong need to affirm that we should be moral. To satisfy this need is to be committed to living a moral life. The need to affirm that we should be moral is so strong that we should satisfy it in this way. Therefore, it is in our self-interest to be moral, and so we have a good reason to be moral.

But what of the conflict between morality and self-interest? We have seen that the demands of morality may come into conflict with the pursuit of self-interest. Since we have argued that it is in our self-interest to be moral, what do we say about this conflict? Aren't we being inconsistent?

There is no real inconsistency here. To see this, let us return to the tire-changing example of section 1: You pass an old man who obviously needs help changing a tire. Since the road is deserted, you are probably the only one who will pass by for a long time. It is inconvenient for you to stop and help since you are already late for dinner at a friend's and you are in a hurry to get there. Still, since the cost to you of stopping to help is just inconvenience, it will maximize happiness in general if you stop and help the old man change his tire. So, morality demands that you put aside your pursuit of self-interest and aid the old man.

This example illustrates the way in which morality and self-interest conflict. The demands of morality conflict with specific plans for pursuing our self-interest, but this does not contradict the fact that it is in our self-interest to be moral. It is in our self-interest to be moral, in the sense that it is in our self-interest to live a certain kind of life, a life based on the general plan of maximizing happiness. It is in our self-interest to hold to this general plan even though it sometimes conflicts with our specific plans. And the reason this is so, we have argued, is that the alternative to the moral life is unsatisfying. In other words, demands of morality may conflict with our specific self-interest (with our specific plans), but even so it is in our general self-interest to be moral (it is in our self-interest to have the general plan of maximizing happiness).

A final word of qualification. We have argued that we should be committed to maximizing happiness in general, and what we have said may have given the impression that this commitment should be total, that the demands of morality should always win out over our specific self-interest. I do not think this is true. Our arguments show that we should have a definite commitment to the moral life. But a definite commitment need not be a total commitment. A definite commitment is compatible with bounds beyond which one will not go. For example, you can be definitely committed to a moral life, yet unwilling to die to maximize happiness in general. But a total commitment would require that you die if that would maximize happiness in general. So, there is always a tension in the moral life between the commitment to morality and the boundaries of that commitment, boundaries that may vary from individual to individual and beyond which specific self-interest reigns.

4. Self-realization, happiness, and freedom

So far we have said that to be moral is to try to maximize happiness in general, and, that it is in our self-interest to have a definite commitment to maximizing happiness in general. But there is one question we have ignored so far: What is happiness? As the ancient Greek philosopher Aristotle points out

> Both the common run of people and cultivated men . . . understand by "being happy" the same as "living well" and "doing well." But when it comes to defining what happiness is, they disagree, and the account given by the common run differs from that of the philosophers. The former say it is some clear and obvious good, such as pleasure, wealth, or honor; some say it is one thing and others another, and often the very same person identifies it with different things at different times.[5]

We will not give a full account of what happiness is; what we will do is identify and explain the essential component of happiness, the component we will call *self-realization*. Self-realization is closely linked to the concept of *freedom,* and one of the main reasons we need to explain self-realization as a component of happiness is to clarify this link to freedom.

To explain self-realization we need to note certain psychological facts. The first is that each of us has an ideal self-image, our conception of how we would most like to be.[6] An ideal self-image is not the same as a self-image. Our self-image is our conception of what we *are* like—not of how we would like to be. Now, we may have more than one ideal self-image, and we may have incompatible ones, but we will have at least one. To simplify matters, we will talk as if each person had just one ideal self-image.

Our ideal self-image is a powerful source of motivation, for we are strongly motivated to act in ways that conform to our ideal self-image. It is easy to see why. What happens if we fail to realize important aspects of our ideal self-image? If we fail to be the way we would most like to be? Clearly, the result will almost always be frustration and unhappiness. An example. Consider a person whom we will call Marcy. It is part of Marcy's ideal self-image to be a painter. Of course, her conception of how she would most like to be will include more than being a painter. But her desire to be a painter is very important to her, and she invests a great deal of time and energy in developing her talent for painting. Now, if in her own eyes she had to regard herself as having failed in her attempt to become a painter, what would be the result? Frustration and unhappiness, certainly; she may even regard her whole life as a failure. On the other hand, if she succeeds she will experience deep pleasure and enjoyment and self-esteem, for that is the typical result of realizing an ideal self-image.

It makes sense then that we are motivated to realize our ideal self-images. And to say this is to say that we are motivated to achieve self-realization, for *self-realization consists in realizing our ideal self-image.* Further, to say that an action realizes part of our ideal self-image is to say two things; first, that the action conforms to, fits with, our ideal self-image; and second, that we perform the action *of our own free will.*[7] The first part of this definition is illustrated by the example of Marcy. But the second part adds something new; that is, the relationship between self-realization and freedom. What is this relationship? We can answer the question by contrasting two examples.

Suppose that you go to medical school because your ideal self-image includes becoming a doctor. Then, going to medical school conforms to your ideal self-image; and if you are going of your own free will, then going to medical school realizes part of your ideal self-image. As a result, you will experience pleasure and enjoyment—assuming that becoming a doctor continues to be part of your ideal self-image and assuming also that you are successful in medical school.[8]

Now, contrast this situation with the following one. Your ideal self-image includes becoming a doctor, but it also includes becoming a biochemist. You realize that you must choose between these two careers since you have not time to pursue both, and so you choose to become a biochemist. But your parents force you, by a combination of financial and emotional pressure, to go to medical school. Here I have in mind an extreme situation in which you are genuinely coerced by all sorts of pressure to alter your plans. In such a case, you do not go of your own free will. (Of course, you could still refuse to go to medical school no matter what the threats, but this fact does not show that you go of your own free will. To go of your own free will is the opposite of being forced, and in this case you were forced. Just as I might force you to hand over all your money by putting a gun to your head. You could still refuse and risk getting killed, but even so it is still true that I forced you to hand over your money; you didn't do it voluntarily—of your own free will.)

Since you do not go to medical school of your own free will, going does *not* realize your ideal self-image—even thought it conforms to it. Of course, your attitude could change while in medical school, and you could end up going of your own free will. But as long as you remain in medical school because you are forced to, going to medical school cannot—by our definition—count as realizing your ideal self-image.

The medical school example helps explain why we have defined self-realization as dependent upon free will. Consider that you will be at least somewhat frustrated and unhappy as long as you remain in medical school only because you are forced to. This is the opposite of the situation in which you go of your own free will. In that case you will experience the pleasure and enjoyment of realizing your ideal self-image. This does not happen in the case in which you are forced to go because then what you are in fact doing conflicts with your conception of what you most want, with your ideal self-image. It is obviously important to distinguish these two sorts of situations since the one involves pleasure and the other, frustration. So, we have defined self-realization in such a way that only the situation in which you act of your own free will counts as self-realization.

These examples illustrate the links between self-realization and the concepts of freedom and happiness. Freedom (acting of your own free will) is, by definition, a necessary condition of self-realization. As for happiness, *self-realization is clearly the essential, central component of happiness, for you cannot be happy unless you realize at least some aspect of your ideal self-image.* The concepts of freedom and happiness have long played a central role in philosophical thought about morality, but they have never before been linked together by the concept of self-realization. And the link is important, for it has two important consequences.

The first consequence is that we try to maximize self-realization in general. This follows from the link with happiness. We have already seen that we should try to maximize happiness in general. Since self-realization is the essential central component of happiness, it follows that we should maximize self-realization in general.

The second consequence is that there is a reason not to interfere with another person's pursuit of those plans and projects which he believes will lead to his self-realization. This follows from the link with freedom. Freedom (acting of your own free will) is a necessary condition of self-realization. Since we should maximize self-realization in general, we have a reason to leave people free—that is, not to interfere with them—when they pursue those plans and projects they believe will lead to their self-realization.

You will notice that the arguments that have led us to recognizing a reason against interfering with people's plans all rest on general facts about people—facts which hold true of people simply and solely by virtue of their being people. We have not appealed to facts about the particular structure of the societies in which people live, nor those that hold just of a single person or a restricted group of people. We have appealed only to the general psychology of people, using facts which hold universally of all persons.

What this means is that our theoretical framework is universal. It is valid for all persons, not just for this or that group or this or that society. In particular, each person—*no matter who he is or what society he lives in*—has a reason not to interfere with another person's plans. Morality demands respect for individual freedom, and it does not restrict this demand to any special group or society. It makes this demand on all persons. So, we can restate the second consequence this way:

> There is a reason why we should not interfere with another person's pursuit of those plans and projects which he believes will lead to his self-realization, *and* each person has this reason simply and solely by virtue of being a person.

We will express this fact by saying that a person has the *right to self-determination*. The following section explains the general concept of a right and examines the implications of the right to self-determination.

5. Rights and the right to self-determination

In discussing morality people often talk about rights without explaining what a right is. This leads to difficulties because people use the word *right* for more than one concept. So, we need to explain what *we* mean by a right. Our concept of a right is based on two ideas. The first idea is that a right is a special kind of reason. Roughly, a person has a right to do X when there is a reason why others should not interfere with his doing X. The second idea is that people have rights simply and solely because they are people. Putting these two ideas together, we get a definition of what a right is:

> A person has a right to do X if and only if there is a reason why others should not interfere with his doing X, and each person has this reason simply and solely because he is a person.

This is what we will mean by a right. It is a convenient term to use in describing various moral issues.

For example, we can now talk of *the right to self-determination*. The right to self-determination is the right to pursue those plans and projects we believe will lead to our self-realization. Given our definition of what a right is, we are justified in speaking of this right, for we saw in the last section that there is a reason why we should not interfere with a person's pursuit of those plans and projects which he believes will lead to his self-realization. And we also saw that each person has this reason simply and solely because he is a person. It is convenient to be able to express this complex fact by speaking of the right to self-determination.

The right to self-determination is the central fact around which we will construct our answers to the practical moral questions we will consider. The issue we will constantly face will be this: when can we justifiably override the right to self-determination? To override (or, as we will sometimes say, to violate) the right to self-determination is to do just what the right says not to do—that is, to interfere with a person's pursuit of those plans and projects which he believes will lead to his self-realization. The question of when we are justified in overriding the right to self-determination constantly arises in practice because people's plans conflict. Take a simple example. Suppose you and I share a car, and suppose that on Saturday you want to drive to the beach while on that same Saturday I want to drive to the mountains. Neither of us wants to stay home. Since you have the right to self-determination, there is a reason why I should not interfere with your plan of going to the beach. But, likewise, since I also have that right, there is a reason why you should not interfere with my plan of going to the mountains. So, how is this situation to be resolved? Since neither of us wants to stay home, we should go one place or the other. But no matter what choice we make, one of us will have his right to self-determination overridden since one of us will have his plans interfered with.

Although in practice there is no way to avoid violating people's rights, this does not mean that we should override a person's right to self-determination whenever it is convenient. There are cases in which we are justified in doing so and others in which we are not. The following example illustrates this point.

Consider a person—let us call him Smith—who is suffering from posttraumatic hydrocephalus. What this means is that, as a result of a blow to the head, Smith has too much spinal fluid. One function of spinal fluid is to fill the space between the brain and the skull; it is like a liquid cushion which protects the brain. Because Smith has too much fluid his brain is being pushed down toward his neck, and this partially pinches off the arteries which supply the brain with blood. As a result Smith suffers from a loss of memory and a loss of reasoning power, plus a number of other disabilities such as lack of coordination. Smith's condition can be dramatically improved by brain surgery. (A shunt is implanted which drains off the excess fluid.) But Smith refuses surgery. In fact, he is vehemently opposed to it; he cannot bear the thought of someone cutting his head open. Smith thinks of having the operation as a sign of weakness and helplessness and refuses because manifesting weakness and helplessness is incompatible with his ideal self-image. So, in avoiding the operation, Smith is pursuing a plan he believes will lead to his self-realization. But Smith's doctor thinks that Smith is not competent to judge whether he should have surgery, and he convinces Smith's wife of this. As a result she goes to court with the doctor and is appointed Smith's legal guardian for the duration of his illness. This gives her the power to force Smith to have the operation, and that is what she does. Smith's wife interferes with her husband's pursuit of a plan he believed would lead to his self-realization, and so she overrides—violates—his right to self-determination. Was she justified in doing this?

The wife is justified. First of all, by avoiding the operation Smith violates his wife's right to self-determination, for certainly his wife is pursuing self-realization by living with him and having his companionship. Smith interferes with her plans by refusing surgery. Not only does this refusal violate his wife's right to self-determination, it also probably makes her profoundly unhappy. So, we are in a situation where we have to weigh the wife's right against the husband's right, and the wife's unhappiness against the husband's opposition to surgery. Basically we are weighing one person's rights and desires against another person's rights and desires. *Whether or not we are justified in overriding the right to self-determination of a particular person in a particular situation depends on whether the balance comes down on the person's side or on our side.* We will discuss many such situations in the chapters which follow, and we will develop some principles for deciding where the balance falls.

In the case of Smith it is pretty clear that the balance falls on the wife's side. Consider that Smith has desires which give him very strong reasons to undergo surgery; among other things Smith desires continued life and health as a mentally competent human being, and this desire can only be satisfied if Smith undergoes surgery. Unfortunately, Smith is suffering from a loss of memory and a loss of reasoning power and does not realize that there is such a good reason for his having surgery. Smith is not rational enough to pursue the course which his own desires give him strong reasons to pursue. It is Smith's irrationality that decides the case against him.

The point is that Smith's irrationality defeats the purpose of leaving Smith free. Why do we leave a person free to act as he wishes? Because freedom is a necessary condition of self-realization, and we should try to maximize self-realization. But when a person is as irrational as Smith is, leaving him free to act as he wishes will definitely not promote self-realization. Smith is so irrational that he chooses plans which are clearly and obviously destructive of his own self-realization as well as his wife's. This is the essential point. Overriding Smith's right to self-determination in this case is justified because Smith's irrationality defeats the purpose of leaving him free, and because his irrationality, if unchecked, would be destructive of his self-realization and his wife's.

Cases involving irrationality are among the most convincing cases in which we can be justified in overriding the right to self-determination, and that is why I have used such a case here as an example. But there are many cases in which we are justified in overriding a person's rights even though the person is not irrational, and we will examine some of these in the chapters that follow.

What the Smith example illustrates is that there is a point to leaving people free until they become extremely irrational. The point is that morality demands we maximize self-realization in general. To do this, we need to leave people free to act as they wish. But extreme irrationality defeats the reason for leaving people free. What we really need to do is leave people free to choose—as long as they make their choices within the limits of rationality.

6. Conclusion: summary of the theoretical framework

There are six basic points by which we can summarize our theoretical framework:

1. It is in our self-interest to be moral. Being moral means being ready (to some degree) to maximize happiness in general.

2. The essential component of happiness is self-realization. Self-realization consists in realizing an ideal self-image. Since we should maximize happiness in general, it follows that we should maximize self-realization in general.

3. Freedom (acting of our own free will) is a necessary condition of self-realization. So, since we should maximize self-realization, there is a reason why we should not interfere with a person's pursuit of those plans and projects he believes will lead to his self-realization. Also, each person has this reason simply and solely because he is a person. We express the fact that this reason exists by saying that people have the right to self-determination.

4. The right to self-determination can be overridden in certain cases. In fact, practical situations always arise in which we need to decide whose right to override. This is an unavoidable consequence of the fact that people's plans conflict.

5. We may be justified or unjustified in overriding a person's right to self-determination. To decide whose right to override we have to

balance the rights and desires of one person against the rights and desires of another.

6. Irrationality can be a factor in justifying us in overriding the right to self-determination. We have a reason to leave people free, but only so long as they make their choices within the limits of rationality. Extreme irrationality makes the pursuit of self-realization ineffective.

NOTES

1. Carl Jung, *Psychological Types* (Princeton, N.J.: Princeton University Press, 1971), p. 212.
2. Søren Kierkegaard, *Either/Or*, trans. David F. Swenson and Lillian Marvin Swenson (Princeton, N.J.: Princeton University Press, 1971), p. 41.
3. This theme has been frequent in modern literature, appearing in works as diverse as Kafka's *The Trial* and Nabokov's *Lolita*. In both life seems unreal and in both I believe the reason can be traced back to the lack of a nonpersonal reason to live.
4. It would be interesting and worthwhile to discuss this point in detail. However, I would like to mention an excellent source of material on these issues—Albert Camus' *The Rebel* (Vintage, 1957), a psychological study of the effects of refusing to affirm that one should be moral.
5. Aristotle, *Nicomachean Ethics*, trans. Martin Ostwald (Indianapolis, Ind.: Bobbs-Merrill, 1962), p. 6.
6. This is a rough explanation. A fuller explanation would go into the issue of how we determine what counts as "most liked."
7. To perform an action of your own free will is, I suggest, for it to be motivated in a certain way by your ideal self-image. We will not develop this idea here, however.
8. Of course, this is a bit simplified. We are assuming that no major tragedies occur in your life like illness or injury.

BIBLIOGRAPHY

Aristotle. *Nicomachean Ethics*, trans. Martin Ostwald. Indianapolis, Ind.: Bobbs-Merrill, 1962.
Williams, Bernard. *Morality*. New York: Harper & Row, 1972.

ONE

Free and Informed Consent

To give consent is to agree. To withhold consent is to refuse to agree. Agreeing and refusing to agree are forms of interaction among people—forms of interaction which are fundamentally important for morality. Why is this sort of interaction so important?

The first point to note is that we do not live solitary, self-sufficient lives isolated from others and independent of them. Rather, each of us depends on others in various ways. In modern societies the division of labor is one major factor which creates this dependence. Take a simple example. A doctor knows how to provide health care but knows little about legal matters; so, to handle such matters, he will have to depend on a lawyer. The lawyer, in turn, will depend on a doctor for health care. Other examples are not hard to find. Just consider that we all depend on the government to do such things as control the economy, maintain law and order, and administer public education, public health care, and welfare. These examples illustrate a fundamentally important fact: *We live in a complex network of social and political relations and dependencies—a network within which each of us traces out his own unique personal history.* This network of social and political organization yields us many advantages. To see this, simply imagine a life stripped of all the advantages that social and political organization confer—schools, markets, homes, museums. Indeed, what would be left? Only a savage and barbaric existence.

But we pay a price for the advantages of social and political organization. We must accept restrictions on our freedom to choose and act as we wish, for effective organization requires that we accept and perform certain roles—even when performing these roles is not what we most want to do. Consider some simple examples. Suppose you are a professor. Your role requires that you give lectures even on days when you would rather do nothing of the sort. Likewise, if you are a surgeon you must show up at the hospital even when you would rather stay home. The point is that—like all of us—the professor and the surgeon buy the advantages of society at the cost of their freedom—not all of their freedom, of course, but some degree of it. This is the price we all pay: The loss of some degree of freedom is the cost of effective social and political organization. Now, there is a danger here, which is that too much freedom may be sacrificed in the name of efficient organization. We should oppose this danger because we need freedom to pursue those plans and projects we believe will lead to self-realization.

There are moral principles on which we can base our opposition to restrictions on our freedom. The right to self-determination is one such principle, but it is not the only one. Another is *the right to give or withhold free and informed consent* to any action which has a significant chance of interfering with those plans and projects we believe will lead to self-realization.[1] For short, we will call this the right to consent. For now, we will just assume that we have this right. Hardly anyone will question this assumption, and, in any case, we will prove later on that our assumption is correct.[2]

How does the right to consent work in practice? Suppose I am suffering from a rare disease for which no effective treatment is known. You are my doctor, and you suggest that a new, experimental drug may be of help. You explain that the drug is dangerous, that it may have serious side effects such as temporary or permanent kidney damage. You do not try to influence my decision about whether to take the drug. You simply place the facts before me for my consideration. After thinking it over, I agree to take the drug. That is, I consent to taking it, for to give consent is to agree. If I had not agreed (either by explicitly refusing or by just remaining silent on the matter), I would have been withholding consent.

Unfortunately, my kidneys are damaged as a result of taking the drug. Are you morally responsible for my injury? Are you morally to blame for it? Surely not. Of course, you did give me the opportunity to take a dangerous drug, but you did so only as a last resort to cure my illness. And you did not force me to take it, or trick me into taking it by withholding information about its dangers. On the contrary, I consented to take it, and my consent was free and informed. It was free because you did not try to influence my decision. If you had pressured me into taking the drug, you would have been morally at fault for my injury because such pressure would have been an unjustifiable infringement on my freedom.

My consent was informed because you informed me about the experimental nature of the drug and, in particular, about its dangers. It would have been wrong to withhold this information from me while offering me the opportunity to take the drug. This would have been an unjustifiable infringement on my freedom, for you would have been deliberately misguiding me by exploiting my trust in you as my doctor.

This example illustrates how the right to consent provides an objective moral ground for opposing infringements of individual freedom. We really do have this right, and actions which violate it without adequate justification are—as a matter of objective fact—morally wrong.

1. Questions and examples

We have seen that the right to consent helps protect individual freedom. If we want to resolve moral dilemmas involving the right to consent we can increase our understanding of this right by asking five fundamental questions. The five answers we give will add up to a single, detailed explanation of how the right to consent protects freedom. The first question is very theoretical while the other four are more practical.

1. *Why do we have the right to consent?* We assumed earlier we had this right, but we have done nothing to justify this assumption. We have done nothing to answer the skeptic who would deny that we have such a right. What would we say to such a person?

We will postpone answering this question until the end of the chapter. But one result of that section must be presented here: a definition of what it is for consent to be informed, since the discussion of the four practical questions that follow will center around the application of this definition to actual situations.

How do we define informed consent? To answer this question, it will be helpful to look at what the California Supreme Court has to say about consent. In 1972 Justice Mosk of California's Supreme Court discussed informed consent in an important and influential decision, *Cobbs* vs. *Grant,* a medical malpractice case. He had to come up with a decision that made good sense in both theory and practice—not an easy thing to do. Justice Mosk stated the essence of his position this way (the references to "the patient" and "the physician" are explained by the fact that this is a medical malpractice case):

> The patient's right of self-decision is the measure of the physician's duty to reveal. *That right can be effectively exercised only if the patient possesses adequate information to enable an intelligent choice.* The scope of the physician's communications to the patient, then, is measured by the patient's need, and that need is whatever information is material to the decision.[3]

There are two points to make about these remarks. First, note that Justice Mosk makes the right to self-determination (or, self-decision, as he says)[4] the cornerstone of his position on consent. This is exactly what we will do, too. When we give our proof that we really do have the right to consent, we will see that the whole point of requiring that consent be informed is to protect the right to self-determination by providing opportunities for free, rational choice. Right now, however, Justice Mosk's second point, italicized in the quoted passage above, is more important for us. This is the idea that a person's consent is informed if he has enough information to make a rational (Mosk says "intelligent") choice. So, if I ask, for example, "How much information do I need to give informed consent to taking an experimental drug?" Justice Mosk's answer is "Enough information about the drug to make a rational decision about whether to take it." This answer is based on a connection between the idea of rational choice and the idea of enough information, and this connection is the key to Mosk's position. The connection between these two ideas can be expressed by saying that *a rational choice must be an informed choice.* More precisely, given several alternatives, a choice of one of them is rational only if that choice is based on a consideration of enough relevant information about the alternatives. A choice not based on such a consideration of relevant information is not a rational choice but at most a guess about which alternative is best.[5] When a person gives informed consent, he has been presented with enough information to make a rational choice as opposed to a guess. His choice may not actually be rational, of course, but he will still have been given the opportunity to make a rational choice.

We can summarize this discussion in the following definition:

A person's giving or withholding consent to an action *A* is informed if and only if that person was presented with enough relevant information about *A* to make a rational choice about whether to do *A*.

A good definition should be useful in practice. To see how our definition fares, let us turn to the four practical questions about the right to consent. We will get a good overview of the practical moral issues raised by consent if we state all the questions at once and illustrate each with an example. We will not try to answer the questions until later. The examples are intended only to illustrate their depth and complexity.

Our first practical question (the second of our five questions) is:

2. *How much information do you need to give informed consent?* Consider the case of Ross, who has been admitted to the hospital with a complaint of severe chest pain. Ross's doctor tells him that he wants to insert a tube into his heart. The doctor explains that he will insert

the tube in an artery in Ross' arm and then push it up and around into his heart. Once the tube is in place, he will inject dye into the heart via the tube; this, he explains, will allow him to take X-rays which will reveal whether certain passageways in Ross's heart have been blocked by fatty deposits of cholesterol. Finding this out, the doctor explains, will enable him to determine whether Ross's condition can be improved by surgery. The doctor also explains there is a very slight risk that the procedure will cause Ross's heart to develop an irregular rhythm, and that if this happens there is a chance Ross might die.

Does Ross have enough information to give or withhold informed consent? He has enough information if he has enough to make a rational choice. But how much is that? This question arises because there is always more relevant information that a person might consider in making a decision. In practice no choice is based on a consideration of all the relevant, available information. For example, in the case of Ross, the dangers of the procedure could have been more fully and accurately described. Ross could have been told that intravascular catheterization with the injection of radio-opaque dye has a 0.01 probability of leading to thrombosis or cardiac arrhythmia. Of course, Ross might not have understood such technical terminology. But does such a lack of understanding excuse us from putting the information before him? Or are we only excused if the information is not needed for a rational decision? And how do we tell what is and is not needed for such a decision? We will consider these questions in section 2.

Our next question about the right to consent is:

3. *How free from the influences of others do you have to be for your consent to be free?* Consider the case of Mr. and Mrs. Jones. Mrs. Jones has just given birth to a child with a serious case of spina bifida. Spina bifida is a birth defect which results from a faulty development of the spinal cord, and in serious cases a sac filled with spinal fluid protrudes from the spinal cord. The child is partially paralyzed; there is a loss of bowel and bladder control and possibly of kidney function. Mental retardation may also occur. Spina bifida can be treated surgically. Without surgery death occurs within a year in 90 percent of the cases. With surgery life expectancy is prolonged, but in serious cases the child will almost certainly be severely handicapped and mentally retarded.

Mr. and Mrs. Jones's doctor presents these facts to them vividly and bluntly, stressing the poor quality of life their child will have even after successful surgery. The doctor wants to be sure he presents the facts about spina bifida accurately and completely, and he is right to be concerned about this. The parents have the right to give or withhold free and informed consent to surgery on their newborn child,[6] and it is the doctor's duty to present them with the information they need.

Mr. and Mrs. Jones consider the facts and finally decide against surgery. The doctor's vivid picture of their child's future misery strongly influenced their decision. Were they so strongly influenced that their decision was not free? Did the blunt and vivid way the doctor informed them of the facts amount to an unjustifiable infringement on their freedom of choice? Perhaps if they had gone to another doctor who was less vivid in conveying the information, they would have decided in favor of surgery. Here the requirement of information conflicts with the requirement of freedom. So, we need to know to what extent we should sacrifice our freedom for the sake of a vivid and detailed presentation of information. And we need especially to know how free from influences a decision must be to count as a free decision. We will take up these issues in section 3.

4. *Under what circumstances, if any, can the right to consent justifiably be violated?* Here let us consider a woman who is a Jehovah's Witness and who needs a blood transfusion to live. Jehovah's Witnesses refuse blood transfusions on religious grounds, and that is what this woman does. She has two small children, and she realizes they will suffer without a mother, but she feels deeply and sincerely that she must remain true to her religious beliefs. So, she withholds consent because, as a Jehovah's Witness, she believes that putting another person's blood in her will defile her body and make it impure. Is her consent informed and free? Can it be informed when she holds religious beliefs which—in the opinion of most of us—make her blind to the actual facts about transfusions and are blatantly irrational? If her consent is not free and informed, would we be justified in violating her right to consent by forcing her to have the transfusion? Or suppose we decide that her consent is indeed both free and informed. Could we still justify violating her right to consent; for example, for the sake of the children? Section 4 considers these questions. We need to arrive at answers that are theoretically and practically sound in order to make choices where people's rights and desires conflict; in this case, the rights and desires of the children conflict with the rights and desires of their mother. This kind of conflict happens constantly, and when it does somebody has to come out the loser, somebody's rights and desires will inevitably be violated. If we want a morality that is useful in practice, we have to know when a violation of a right is justified, and when it is not.

5. *What principles govern consenting in another's behalf?* It is sometimes impossible for a person to give free and informed consent. For

example, you cannot give or withhold consent if you are taken unconscious to the emergency room after an auto accident. Suppose this happens to you, and suppose the surgeon wants to amputate your severely injured leg. He asks me—your brother—to consent to this operation on your behalf. This is the usual practice. The patient's spouse, legal guardian, or closest living available relative is asked to act as the patient's proxy and give or withhold consent on the patient's behalf. But when is such proxy consent informed? I know what it is for my consent to be informed when I am consenting for myself, but what information do I need when I am acting as your proxy, consenting for you? Should I consider what you might do? Or should I just pay attention to what the surgeon thinks is medically best? How should I act in order to best protect your freedom? We will consider proxy consent in section 5. It is an extremely important topic, for what we say about proxy consent will partially determine what we will say about euthanasia, abortion, infanticide, the rights of mental patients, and the rights of children.

If we answer questions (2)-(5), we will have a full and detailed answer to the question of how the right to consent functions in actual practice to protect individual freedom. We will take each question in turn.

2. When is consent informed?

How much information do we need to give informed consent? We know that our consent is informed if we have been presented with enough information to provide us with the opportunity to make a rational decision. But how much is enough? In the case of Ross there is a good deal more information he could have been given if his medical knowledge had been greater. Then precise medical terminology could have been used to describe the relevant facts with more completeness and detail than was actually possible. A complete and detailed set of facts is indeed relevant to making a rational choice. So, shouldn't we at least attempt to convey them to Ross? He will not understand much of what we say, but does that excuse us?

Yes, it does. What sense would it make to use precise terminology which Ross will not understand? No sense at all. The whole point of presenting Ross with the information is to enable him to make a rational choice, and we obviously cannot enable him to do that by presenting facts to him in a way he will find unintelligible. When we present information to a person prior to his giving consent, we must present that information in language the person can understand. In the case of medical treatment, for example, it is up to the doctor to decide how to best present the relevant facts. In making this decision the doctor must weigh completeness and accuracy against intelligibility. Usually, as in the case of Ross, this will mean that the doctor will have to sacrifice some degree of completeness and precision for the sake of intelligibility.

In determining how to work out a compromise between completeness and intelligibility, we must use our own judgment. There is no strict set of rules we can use to decide how to make this compromise. In this area the moral sensitivity and practical wisdom of the individual cannot be replaced by any impersonal procedure. This is an especially important point to stress in the case of medical treatment. Doctors—or other health-care professionals involved in treating patients—are not just competent technicians treating the body. They must also adequately inform their patients of what they are doing, and this requires that they bring to the fore their moral sensitivity and practical wisdom.

Now, let us turn again to what the courts have to say about informed consent. Justice Mosk, in his decision in *Cobbs* vs. *Grant,* agrees with what we have said about the need to compromise between completeness and accuracy, and intelligibility. It is his opinion that

> the patient's interest in information does not extend to a lengthy polysyllable discourse on all possible complications. A mini-course in medical science is not required; the patient is concerned with the risk of death or bodily harm, and problems of recuperation.[7]

He then makes the additional point that

> there is no physician's duty to discuss the relatively minor risks inherent in common procedures, when it is common knowledge that such risks inherent in the procedure are of very low incidence.[8]

Justice Mosk illustrates this point by noting that the risks inherent in taking a blood sample include hemotoma, dermititis, cellulitis, abcess, osteomyelitis, septicemia, endocarditis, thrombophlebitis, pulmonary embolism, and death. His point is that, since it is common knowledge in the medical profession that these complications are extremely unlikely, your doctor is not required to inform you of them. Mosk concludes that

> when there is a common procedure a doctor must, of course, make such inquiries as are required to determine if for the particular patient the treatment under consideration is contraindicated—for example, to determine if the patient has had adverse reactions to antibiotics—

but no warning beyond such inquiries is required as to the remote possibility of death or serious bodily harm.[9]

Justice Mosk's position makes good sense. To see why, consider again our definition of informed consent. We said that consent is informed when the person has been presented with enough information to make a rational choice. However, when the probability of a risk is very low, you do not need to take it into account in making a rational decision. Each time you cross even a quiet, residential street there is still a very slight risk of being hit by a car. But because the risk is so slight, you do not worry about it. And rightly so. Likewise, there is no point to worrying about minor risks involved in routine medical procedures. As we noted above, it is possible to die as a result of complications following the taking of a common blood sample. But no (rational) person worries about this, and your doctor is not required to mention the possibility to you. He has to give you enough information to enable you to make a rational decision, but he does not need to mention such very minor risks because risks like that simply do not need to be considered. In general, then, consent can be informed even when very minor risks have not been mentioned.

So far we have been saying there are certain things we do not need to do when we present information to a person prior to his giving consent. However, when the risks involved are not minor, there are certain items of information that must be presented if consent is to be informed. Suppose, for example, that we want Smith to consent to test pilot the new, one-person, jet-powered mini-helicopter we have invented. We are not sure it will fly, so there are risks involved that are certainly not minor. Here we must inform Smith of two things. First, we must describe the essentials of what we want him to do. How high do we want him to fly? Where do we want him to fly? What maneuvers do we want him to perform? And so on. Second, we must describe the risks involved. We must, for example, tell him what we estimate the likelihood of a crash to be. If we do not have any idea of how likely a crash is, then we must tell him so.

Unless we inform Smith on these two points, he will not have enough information to make a rational decision. Of course, depending on the situation, there may be still more that we should tell Smith. For example, if we intend our helicopter to be used as a highly destructive military weapon, it may be that we should tell Smith so, for this piece of information might greatly influence his decision about whether to test the machine. But there are no fixed rules which will always tell us how much information we must impart; rather, we will have to rely on our judgment.

Generalizing from our discussion of Smith, we can say that a person's consent to an action *A* is informed only if that person has been presented (in language he can understand) with (1) a description of the essentials of the proposed action *A*, and (2) a description of the (non-minor) risks inherent in the action *A*. What counts as a "description of the essentials" will vary from case to case. *In medical treatment it should include a description of any alternative treatments which are genuinely feasible options and an explanation of why the particular treatment proposed was chosen.* The reason for this is that patients are almost totally dependent on the knowledge and judgment of their doctors, and cannot be expected to know about feasible alternatives or reasons for preferring one to another. So, if they are to make a rational choice for or against a proposed treatment, they should be informed about these alternatives and the reasons for choosing one as opposed to another. This does not mean that the patient must be given a "mini-course in medical science," for it is almost always possible to explain a proposed treatment in terms that are both plain and accurate.

In conclusion, the rationale for requiring that consent be informed is to protect the right to self-determination by giving people the opportunity to make free, rational choices. This rationale is based on the fact that a rational choice must be an informed choice. Getting the relevant information across to the person who is to give consent, however, often poses practical problems. One problem is the conflict between the requirement that consent be informed and the requirement that it be free. We gave an example of this conflict in our discussion of the question: How free from the influences of others do we have to be for our consent to be free? It is time now to take up that question in detail and to investigate the conflicts which arise between the requirement of information and the requirement of freedom.

3. When is consent free?

There is no simple answer to our third question. We can approach it by taking note of various facts about the concept of freedom. The most basic fact is simply that freedom is important. Justice Mosk insists on this in his decision in *Cobbs* vs. *Grant*. A patient, he claims, has the

> basic right ... to make the ultimate informed decision regarding the course of treatment to which he knowledgeably consents to be subjected.
>
> A medical doctor, being the expert, appreciates the risks inherent in the procedure he is prescribing, the risks of a decision not to undergo treatment, and the probability of a successful outcome

of the treatment. But once this information has been disclosed, that aspect of the doctor's expert function has been performed. *A weighing of these risks against the individual subjective fears and hopes of the patient is not an expert skill. Such evaluation and decision is a nonmedical judgment reserved to the patient alone.* A patient should be denied the opportunity to weigh the risks only where it is evident he cannot evaluate the data, as for example, where there is an emergency or the patient is a child or incompetent. .... In all cases other than the foregoing, the decision whether or not to undertake treatment is vested in the party most directly affected: the patient.[10]

Mosk tells us in no uncertain terms that the individual's freedom to choose must be respected. His reason is that the person who is to give consent is in the best possible position to weigh the risks involved against his own "individual subjective fears and hopes." This certainly is true. Nobody but me possesses my own subjective point of view; I can see into my own mind, see my own hopes, fears, desires, and beliefs in a way no one else can. But there is also a deeper reason why people should be left free: We should leave people free to choose as they wish because *the exercise of free choice is a necessary condition of self-realization.*

Now, what does this requirement mean? What makes a choice free? Since many people find the idea of free choice (acting of your own free will) a puzzling one, we should explain what we mean here. Intuitively we tend to think of a free choice as one which is "internally" motivated as opposed to "externally" motivated. To see what is correct in this intuitive idea, contrast these two situations. In the first, you read all of Nabokov's novels simply because it is part of your ideal self-image to be well acquainted with Nabokov's works. In the second, you also read them all, but this time you do so because—and only because—they were assigned in a course you are taking. In the first situation your reading the novels is "internally" motivated; it is motivated by your ideal self-image, and it is motivated "directly" because your ideal self-image includes being well acquainted with Nabokov's works. But in the second situation your motivation is clearly "external" since you are reading the novels only because they were assigned for the course. Now, your ideal self-image may include doing well in the course you are taking, and this may be what motivates you to read the novels. But in this case the connection between your ideal self-image and motivation is less "direct," and the motivation more a result of external circumstances.

If we wanted to give a full account of free choice, we would have to say a good deal more about what an ideal self-image is, and we would, of course, have to explain fully the distinction between direct and indirect motivation. These would be interesting issues to pursue, but they would lead us far away from the practical moral problems raised by the right to consent. In practice there are various sources of indirect motivation a person must deal with. In medical cases the chief sources include the patient's family and friends as well as the hospital staff. Economic factors may also play a role. In such cases the degree of freedom of a choice is determined by (1) the extent to which it is directly motivated by the person's ideal self-image, and (2) the extent to which the choice is not influenced by the indirect sources of motivation—family, friends, the hospital staff, and economic considerations.

Ideally, then, a person who is to give consent should be presented with the relevant information and left completely free to make up his mind. But in practice this will never happen. In practice the very act of presenting information influences the person's decision, and this means the decision cannot possibly be completely free. We illustrated this point in the last section with the case of Mr. and Mrs. Jones, for we saw that *the way* in which their doctor presented the information about spina bifida had a strong effect on their decision.

To what extent, then, should we sacrifice freedom for the sake of information? And, exactly how free from the influences of others should a decision be? These questions raise both theoretical and practical issues. On the theoretical side we need a better understanding of the nature of freedom. On the practical side we need a guideline which gives us some indication of how to balance an increase in the forcefulness and effectiveness with which information is presented against a decrease in freedom.

To begin with theory, the first point to note is that we are free to choose to do as we wish—to a degree. *Freedom is always a matter of degree,* because when we make a choice we are almost always influenced by others in many different ways.[11] Other people may give us advice, point out relevant facts, or threaten us, or they may influence us simply because we are concerned about what they will think. Of course, the degree to which we are under the influence of others varies greatly. If you order me at gunpoint to open the door, I have very little choice but to do as you say—if I want to live—so I am greatly under your influence. If, on the other hand, you casually mention that I might open the door, I may not be influenced by you at all. Still, we should not think we can make choices which are completely free, uninfluenced by others in any way at all. This is an ideal we can approach but never reach. The most we can do is strive to make our choices as free as possible. This applies to consent. Giving or withholding consent should be as free as possible in the circumstances.

From a practical point of view, what we want is a guideline which will aid us in determining when the giving or withholding of consent is "as free as possible in the circumstances." We can reason our way to the right guideline. Consider first that our goal is to make your giving or withholding consent as free as possible. But we know we will influence you when we present the relevant information to you. We cannot avoid this since we must make your consent informed. So, to keep your choice as free as possible, we should (a) try to make sure that we do not influence you in any other way besides presenting the information, and (b) present the information in a way that is "neutral"— that reflects as little personal bias as possible for one alternative as opposed to another. We can illustrate the guideline expressed in (a) and (b) by returning to the case of Mr. and Mrs. Jones.

Mr. and Mrs. Jones's doctor acted in accord with (a). He did not, for example, express his own opinion about whether surgery should be performed. This would have been a clear violation of (a) and an unjustifiable attempt to infringe on the freedom of the parents. But did the doctor act in accord with (b)? This is the difficult question. He presented a vivid picture of the life of a spina bifida child. He did this because he wanted the parents to grasp fully what they would be doing if they opted for surgery. But did he go too far? He wanted to give accurate information, but did the way in which he gave this information reflect— perhaps unintentionally—a bias in favor of refusing surgery? There is no simple answer here. The doctor is confronted with a difficult task. He wants to get the information across to the parents, and a vivid, forceful picture of spina bifida is a good tool to use for this purpose. Unfortunately, a vivid, forceful picture can capture the imagination and bias a person in favor of one choice as opposed to another, and the doctor must also aim at keeping the parents' choice as free as possible. The only solution is to compromise, to strike a balance between an effective presentation of the information and a presentation that leaves the parents as free as possible. Again, we must be guided by our own personal judgment, by our own moral sensitivity and practical wisdom, for we will never find a set of rules that will decide these matters for us.

4. Overriding the right to consent

In what circumstances, if any, are we justified in overriding someone's right to consent? Let us turn to the Jehovah's Witness example we considered earlier.

To repeat, a woman who is a Jehovah's Witness needs a blood transfusion. She realizes that her husband and her two small children—none of whom are themselves Jehovah's Witnesses—will suffer, but she feels deeply and sincerely that she must remain true to her religious beliefs. Should we respect the woman's right to consent and let her die as a result of refusing the transfusion? Or should we override her right and save her life by forcing her to have the transfusion? This is a case in which people are in conflict, and there is no simple answer because this conflict cannot be resolved without violating at least one person's rights and frustrating his or her desires. Still, this particular conflict can be resolved, and it is useful to see how, for by doing so we will arrive at a general answer to our question about when we can justifiably override the right to consent.

We need to look at the situation more closely, and the first question to ask is whether the woman's consent is informed and free. It is informed provided that she was presented with enough information to make a rational decision. *Presented* is the crucial word here. We may suppose that her doctor explained to her all the relevant facts about the blood transfusion. But given that she has religious beliefs which, in the opinion of most of us, blind her to the actual facts, can we really hold that she was presented with the facts? The situation is like trying to present a gift to someone who keeps turning his back on you and refusing to even acknowledge your attempt to give it. Now, if the woman's consent could not possibly be informed, then she could not make a rational choice. And if she cannot, then we might be justified in stepping in and making the decision for her.

But is her consent informed or not? I think the woman's consent is informed. She was presented with the information. What is required for a presentation of the information is that she understand what is said to her. If she ignores or disbelieves what she has heard and understood, that is her prerogative. As long as she comprehends what is said, and consequently has the opportunity to accept and use the information, her consent is informed. Now, there are many cases in which a person really is incapable of understanding the information that would have to be presented for his consent to be informed. Such cases raise important issues, and we will consider them in section 5.

We have decided the woman's consent is informed, but is it free? She is under the sway of religious beliefs which—in the minds of most of us—are blatantly irrational. Is consent free when it is influenced by a powerful but irrational religious conviction? If we decide that her consent is not free, we might also decide that we should violate her right to consent by forcing her to have the transfusion. After all, it is sometimes right to forcibly save a person from the consequences of acting on an irrational compulsion. For example, if you were suddenly seized by the wild impulse to jump out the window of the top-floor apartment of a high-rise, I certainly ought to grab you and stop you. No doubt you would be more than grateful to me once the impulse had passed.

So, should we interfere with the woman's decision on the ground that her consent is not free, or is it really free after all? The answer, I think, is that her consent is free enough. We all have fundamental beliefs which guide us as we trace out our unique individual histories; and even though they guide us, this does not mean those beliefs thereby deprive us of our freedom. Rather, they are part of that which makes us what we are. A basic belief can, of course, become too influential. Consider, for example, the mentally disordered person who believes he is God and who steps in front of a truck to prove he will not be hurt. But the woman we are considering is quite competent mentally, and she is not at the mercy of her religious beliefs in the way a mentally disordered person is at the mercy of his fantasies and delusions. So her withholding of consent is free, or at least free enough since freedom is always a matter of degree.

But are there other grounds on which we can justify overriding the woman's right to consent, even though we grant that her withholding of consent is free and informed? The answer is yes. The woman's rights and desires are not the only thing we have to consider. There are three other factors we must also take into account: her family, her relationship with her doctor, and her duties to society as a whole. When we take all the relevant factors into consideration, we will see that we can—in this particular case—justify overriding her right to consent by forcing her to have the transfusion. Let us consider the various factors one at a time.

First, there is the family. Both the woman's husband and her children have the right to self-determination—the right to pursue those plans and projects they believe will lead to self-realization. Now, while neither the husband nor the children are very likely to use the term *self-realization* to express their beliefs, the husband believes his wife is important to him in a particular way, and the children believe their mother is important to them in a particular way. It is this particular way which we call "leading to self-realization." If we decide we must respect the woman's right to consent and let her die, we will be acting in a way that interferes with the right to self-determination of the husband and children. Of course, if we decide to respect their right to self-determination, we will force the transfusion on the woman and thus override her right to consent. Somebody's right is going to be overridden no matter what. Whose should it be?

We should not try to answer this question until we have taken all the relevant factors into account, and the next factor to consider is the woman's relationship with her doctor. Let us suppose the woman entered the hospital voluntarily and placed herself under medical care of her own free will, and while she refuses the blood transfusion, she does wish to remain in the hospital under professional medical care. There is a conflict here. The doctor's professional standards require him to perform the routine procedure of a blood transfusion for his patient; that is the treatment which is medically indicated. But if he is to respect the woman's wishes, he must act counter to his own professional standards, counter to his professional goal of saving life. By asking the doctor to act counter to this goal, the woman is interfering in an important way with the doctor's right to self-determination.

Finally, let us turn to society as a whole. Society—the complex network of social and political organization in which we live—has an interest in ensuring that children are well-cared for. Well-cared-for children are more likely to be successful and to contribute to the economic, political, and cultural advance of society than poorly cared-for children. Since the woman lives in and benefits from the network of social and political organization, it makes sense to say that she owes something in return, and certainly one thing she owes is caring for her children adequately. If we think she should be allowed to choose to die as a result of refusing the transfusion, we must explain why she should be freed from the debt she owes society as a whole. I do not mean to imply that we could not come up with such an explanation; I just want to point out that what the woman owes society is one more factor to take into consideration.

Now we have considered all the relevant factors, what can we say about whose rights should be overridden? We can make a strong case that the woman should be forced to have the transfusion. If we force her to have it, we protect the rights and desires of the husband, the two children, and the doctor, and we act in accord with the interest of society as a whole. If we let her die, we protect her right at the cost of violating the rights and frustrating the desires of four others, as well as acting in a socially counterproductive way. In this particular case the balance comes down on the side of transfusion. If the case were different, if—for example—she had no children, our decision might very well be different.

What we have done here is weigh the rights and desires of one individual against the rights and desires of four others and the interests of society as a whole. What principles guided us in weighing these factors? We implicitly followed two guidelines: (1) minimize the number of rights violated; and (2) maximize the number of desires satisfied. These are the guidelines we should follow in resolving cases of conflict among rights; they will help us determine when a right can be justifiably overridden. The guidelines are justified as a means of leading us to act in the way that is most conducive to the self-realization (and freedom) of the greatest number of people.

But we should emphasize that they are only guidelines. They should not be applied mechanically. For example, consider what we would do if the woman's children were almost fully grown; while they would greatly miss their mother, they would still function and develop adequately without her. In such a case I think we should respect the woman's right to consent and let her die, even though doing so conflicts with both our guidelines.

The fact that our guidelines cannot be applied mechanically should not trouble us unduly. Even though we lack explicit rules to decide all cases, we do nonetheless weigh rights and desires against each other and are able to make decisions. We argue over decisions, sometimes agreeing eventually, sometimes not. This is a part of human life. The lack of rules will bother those who think that something does not make sense unless it is codifiable or quantifiable. But aren't such people overlooking the fact that in daily life we must make sense of and deal with moral dilemmas without recourse to rules?[12]

One final point remains. Even though we have concluded that we should override the woman's right to consent, it is definitely not permissible for us to go ahead and force the blood transfusion on her. We have to first go to court and obtain a legal order. In complex cases like this one, the court is the proper place to resolve a conflict of rights and desires, for it is a nonpartisan institution which can consider all the relevant factors and take into account anything that makes the particular case before it an exception to the guidelines we gave above. This ensures the fairest treatment of all concerned.

It is worth summarizing the main points we have made in this section. There are three. First, a person's right, such as his right to consent, may sometimes be justifiably overridden in cases where that person's exercise of his right conflicts with the rights and desires of others.[13] Second, in deciding whether we are justified in overriding someone's right we should follow the guidelines of minimizing the number of rights violated and maximizing the number of desires satisfied. Third, in many cases the courts are the proper place to resolve conflicts of people's rights and desires.

5. Proxy consent

What principles govern consenting in another's behalf? The issue of proxy consent—consenting in another's behalf—arises when the person we would normally ask to give free and informed consent cannot do so. This happens in three cases: with people who are unconscious, with people who are suffering from a mental disorder so severe that their giving or withholding of consent would not be free or informed, and with children who are too immature to give or withhold consent in a truly free and informed way.

Let us reconsider the case in which you are taken unconscious to the emergency room after an auto accident. The surgeon wants to amputate your leg, which is severely injured, and he asks me—your brother—to consent to this operation in your behalf. What should I do?

I think the answer is clear. I should figure out what you would do if you could give free and informed consent, and then I should make that choice for you. If I approached the situation in any other way, I would run the risk of interfering with those plans and projects you believe *will lead to your self-realization.* I would therefore be running the risk of interfering with your right to self-determination, and there is nothing in the situation which justifies me in taking that risk. The points we have just made can be conveniently summarized in the following principle:

> (P1) A person *x* ought to give consent to an action *A* on behalf of another person *y* if and only if *x* has good reason to think that *y* would give free and informed consent to *A* if *y* were able to give or withhold free and informed consent.

(P1) applies only in certain cases. These are cases in which this condition holds: the person who is to give or withhold consent in another person's behalf knows enough about that person to be able to figure out with a high degree of certainty what that person would do if he were able to give free and informed consent.

What happens when this condition is not fulfilled? Suppose you have arrived unconscious in the emergency room after an auto accident, but this time there is no one available who knows you. The surgeon thinks he should amputate your leg, but now there is no one whom he can ask to give or withhold consent in your behalf. What should he do? You will die, or at best suffer severe and dangerous complications, if he does not amputate. The surgeon does not want to run these risks; he insists that, from a medical point of view, amputation is a necessity—and it must be performed immediately. There is no time to wait until you become conscious.

The best advice we can give the surgeon is to go ahead and amputate. This is the action most likely to be in accord with your plans for self-realization. We do not know what your plans are, but whatever they are it is very likely that you can only successfully realize them if you continue life as a physically and mentally healthy human being. So, the surgeon should act in the way that has the best chance of maintaining your physical and mental health. This means amputation. This course of action is justified as the one most likely to be compatible with your plans for self-realization and least likely to interfere with your freedom and your right to self-determination.

We can extract a general principle from this example. Consider what is essential to it. There are two people, x and y. One of them, x (the surgeon), is in a position to perform an action A (amputating the leg) which is, in all probability, necessary to maintain the health of the other person, y. But y is unconscious and no one is available to give proxy consent. In addition, the situation is an emergency since the action A (amputation) should not be delayed. In such a situation the following principle applies:

(P2) With respect to y, x should perform those therapeutic actions— and *only* those therapeutic actions—which are, in all probability, necessary to maintain y's physical and mental health.[14]

By following this principle we will act in the way that is least likely to interfere with individual freedom and the right to self-determination. As we will see in the next two chapters, (P2) has important implications for the issues of euthanasia, abortion, and infanticide.

So far (P2) applies only in cases involving people who are unconscious, who are in an emergency situation, and so on. However, this principle can also be extended to cover certain cases involving children. Consider this case, for example. A nine-year-old boy is suffering from a chronic kidney disease. To live, he requires frequent dialysis. This means he is connected to a machine (the dialysis machine) which cleanses his blood, a function his kidneys can no longer perform. The connection is accomplished by tubes inserted in his veins—one tube to take the blood out, one to put it back in. Patients who require frequent dialysis over a long period of time occasionally refuse to continue with it—even though they know this means death. For some people the experience of dialysis is simply psychologically and physically intolerable. The nine-year-old boy in our example decides he is one of these people, and he refuses to continue dialysis. He says he would rather die.

(P2) applies in this case. To see how, we first need to determine whether the boy's withholding of consent is free and informed. For the purposes of our example, let us suppose that we decide it is informed but not free. We are convinced that he understands he will die and that he grasps the reality of his own death, so his withholding of consent is informed. But we also become convinced that his decision is not free. What convinces us is the discovery that his decision was strongly influenced by an adult patient whom the boy admired and idolized. This patient refused further dialysis earlier in the week, and the boy knew of his decision and had even discussed it with him. When we talk with the boy we find that he is very depressed at the thought that the man will die, and we become convinced that he is dealing with his depression by trying to live up to the example of the man he idolized. In light of these facts we decide that his decision was not free (that is, the degree of freedom involved was very low). We also decide that this boy under these circumstances is not *capable* of giving or withholding free and informed consent to further dialysis. Since he is not capable of making a free and informed decision, we are not morally required to go along with his decision to refuse dialysis.[15]

But what should we do? Maybe the boy really does find dialysis intolerable. This could be true even if his actual decision to discontinue dialysis was strongly influenced by the example of the adult patient. So, what should we do about this possibility? That depends on who we are. If we are the boy's doctors, it is wrong for us to make a decision like this for the boy. After all, he is a person with rights like the right to self-determination and the right to consent. We must respect these rights.

The responsibility for deciding what to do falls on the parents. Since they brought him into existence, they are responsible for caring for him until he can care for himself. So what should the parents do? What principle should guide them in giving proxy consent here? They should follow (P1) if it applies, for this is the course that will best protect their child's right to self-determination. But (P1) applies only if the parents are in a position to determine what their child would do if he were able to give free and informed consent, and the parents may not be in a position to determine this. The reason they may not is that a child does not have a fully developed personality, and the lack of a fully developed personality may in some cases make it impossible to figure out what the child would do if he were able to give free and informed consent. To figure out what the boy would do, we have to consider his personality—his beliefs, desires, traits, and attitudes—and ask: What would someone with this personality choose if he could make a free and informed choice? But, in the case of a child this question may often be impossible to answer because his attitudes—toward death, the value of life, the pain of psychological stress, his parents' feelings for him, and his feelings toward his parents—are still being formed; his personality is still being developed.

For the sake of our example, let us suppose (P1) does not apply for these reasons. Then the parents should follow (P2), for this ensures the least interference with their child's present and, more importantly, with his future, mature plans for self-realization. Now, following (P2) does not necessarily mean that the parents should consent to further dialysis. According to (P2) they should act in ways that maintain or promote the boy's health. But promoting health is not always the same as prolonging life. If the boy really does find dialysis intolerable, if he would really prefer to die, then it is possible that the way to promote his health is to discontinue dialysis. We will not argue for this point until Chapter 2; what we want to point out here is the fact that (P2) does not tell us what to decide; rather, it tells us what to consider in making our decision.

Children do have rights. We cannot think their rights are easily over-ridden simply because they are sometimes incapable of making a free and informed decision. For example, suppose the boy in our example was sixteen instead of nine. Would we be justified in overriding his refusal to continue dialysis? There is a fairly well-known case in which a sixteen-year-old girl refused further dialysis and was allowed to die.[16]

By now perhaps it is not necessary to mention that (P1) and (P2) are not strict rules but just guidelines to which there can be justifiable exceptions. Take (P2), for example. Some people hold that (P2) can be justifiably violated when it is necessary to use large numbers of children to test a new, experimental vaccine.[17] Rubella vaccine was tested on retarded children living in special care centers. The supervising adults gave proxy consent for the children—in violation of (P2) since testing the vaccine *risked* the children's health rather than promoted it. Some people argue that the possible good to be derived from the vaccine justified the violation of (P2). We will not try to decide whether this claim is correct. The point we want to make is that this is the kind of situation in which the question of overriding (P2) can legitimately be raised.

We have not yet said anything about proxy consent in the case of people who are suffering from a mental disorder so severe that they are incapable of giving or withholding free or informed consent. We can override the right to consent of such people.[18] But what principles should guide us here? It turns out that neither (P1) nor (P2) is entirely appropriate. This question is both important and complex and we will devote Chapter 4 to examining it.

6. Conclusion

We now have a fairly good picture of how the right to consent works in practice. Throughout, we have emphasized that working with the right to consent is not a matter of applying strict rules but of using our personal judgment and moral sensitivity. This emphasis reflects the fact that our moral perspective insists on the importance of the individual and his or her capabilities for free choice and rational judgment. It is easy to lose sight of the importance of individual human lives and, as a result, to lose sight of the importance of the moral constraints which the right to consent imposes on human interaction. The world contains millions of people interacting in extremely complex patterns. Viewed from this perspective, does it really matter much whether we respect a given individual's right to consent in a particular situation? In the long run what difference will it make? We must resist such disillusioning thoughts. As the psychoanalyst Carl Jung writes:

> In the face of huge numbers every thought of individuality pales, for statistics obliterate everything unique. Contemplating such overwhelming might and misery, the individual is embarrassed to exist at all. Yet the real carrier of life is the individual. He alone feels happiness, he alone has virtue and responsibility and any ethics whatever. The masses and the state have nothing of the kind.[19]

THEORETICAL FOUNDATIONS

It is now time to return to our first question about the right to consent: Why do we have the right to consent? We will answer this by deriving the right to consent from the right to self-determination; that is, we will show that, given this assumption (which we proved earlier)[20], we can prove we have the right to consent. Besides proving this, the derivation will also illuminate the relation between the right to consent and freedom. We will see that the right to consent protects freedom by protecting the right to self-determination.

A derivation, or proof, starts from an assumption and proceeds step by step to the conclusion. Our derivation begins with the assumption that we have the right to self-determination, and it will take us four steps to get from that assumption to the conclusion that we have the right to consent. The first step is one that we have already taken. In the Introduction we discussed the right to self-determination, and we saw that *we each have good reason to ensure that people have the greatest possible opportunity to make and carry out free, rational choices.*[21] The italicized sentence expresses the first step in our derivation. This step takes us from the right to self-determination to the idea of maximizing free, rational choice.

The second step links the idea of free, rational choice to the idea of informed choice; it is that *a rational choice must be an informed choice.* More precisely, given several alternatives a choice of one of them is rational only if that choice is based on a consideration of (enough) relevant information about the alternatives. A choice not based on such a consideration of relevant information is not a rational choice but at best a guess about which alternative is best.

We can now conclude that we have good reason to ensure that people have the greatest possible opportunity to make and carry out free and informed choices. Why? Because a rational choice must be an informed choice, and we have good reason to maximize the opportunities for making and carrying out free, rational choices.

This brings us to our third step. This step links the idea of consent to the idea of choice by pointing out that *to give or withhold consent is to make a choice.* Now, we have just seen that we have good reason to ensure that people have the greatest possible opportunity to make free and informed choices. But since to give or withhold consent is to make a choice, it follows that we have good reason to ensure that people have the greatest possible opportunity to give or withhold free and informed consent. We also have good reason to ensure that their giving or withholding of consent is not overridden. This follows because we have good reason to maximize the opportunities for making and carrying out free and informed choices. This point is not inconsistent with the fact that we are sometimes justified in overriding a person's right to consent. In the Jehovah's Witness case, for example, we do have a reason to respect the woman's right to consent. But we have a better, stronger reason to override it.

Our fourth and final step consists in showing that the fact that we each have this reason means we have the right to consent. Recall how we defined what a right is:[22]

A person *x* has a right to do *y* if and only if there is a reason why others should not interfere with *x*'s doing *y*, and each person has this reason simply by virtue of the fact that he is a person.

We have the right to give or withhold free and informed consent, then, if and only if

there is a reason why others should not interfere with another person's giving or withholding of consent, and each person has this reason simply by virtue of being a person.

Does such a reason exist? It does. We saw in the third step that we each have good reason to maximize the opportunities for giving or withholding free and informed consent. We also have good reason to ensure that the giving or withholding of consent is not overridden. The less we interfere, the more we maximize the opportunities to give or withhold consent; and the less we interfere, the more we ensure that the giving or withholding of consent will not be overridden. Thus there is a reason why others should not interfere with a person's giving or withholding of free and informed consent.

Does each person have this reason simply by virtue of being a person? A look back over our reasoning here will show that the answer is *yes*. At no point do we appeal to any fact which does not hold of all people at all times simply by virtue of their being people.

So, we have our conclusion: we do have the right to consent. We have also seen the connection between the right to consent and the right to self-determination. By respecting the right to consent, we help maximize the opportunities for free, rational choice. Making free, rational choices is a necessary condition of achieving self-realization. So, by respecting the right to consent, we safeguard individual freedom and the right to self-determination. Limitations on our freedom interfere with our rights. When we respect the right to consent, we help maximize the opportunities for making free, rational choices. So, respecting the right to consent protects individual freedom and the right to self-determination. Finally, it is worth pointing out the second and third steps of the derivation establish a connection between informed consent and rational choice. It is this connection which shows the correctness of the definition of informed consent which we gave earlier.

FURTHER QUESTIONS

There are many questions about the right to consent which we have not discussed. Here are four I think it useful to consider.

1. Mr. Smith and Mr. Jones are both hospitalized with the same disease. Mr. Jones is a rather unintelligent and poorly educated man. He has no desire to know about his disease; he just wants to get cured and get out of the hospital. Still, he has the right to consent,

and so his doctors must present to him a certain minimal amount of information. Mr. Smith, on the other hand, is intelligent and well-educated, and wants to know about his disease and what the doctors are doing. He is quite capable of understanding lengthy and complicated explanations. Are Mr. Smith's doctors morally required to present Mr. Smith with more than the minimal amount of information that was presented to Mr. Jones? If so, should Mr. Jones have been presented with this information also?

2. Consent should be free and informed. But we often sacrifice a certain degree of freedom for the sake of greater information, as we saw in section 3. Are there cases in which the sacrifice goes the other way—where we sacrifice information for the sake of freedom?

3. Can you describe a case in which a Jehovah's Witness refuses a blood transfusion and in which he should be allowed to die as a result?

4. I am a professional racing car driver who has just suffered a nearly fatal accident. I have been rushed unconscious to the nearest hospital. There the surgeon asks you—my sister—to consent to the amputation of both my legs. Unless the legs are amputated my chances of surviving are very low. What do you do? I have often said that if I could not race, I would rather die. And I have also often said that I would rather die than survive as a cripple after a racing accident. Your problem is that you do not know how seriously I meant these things. If I were conscious and really faced with death, would I choose to die? How would you deal with this situation?

NOTES

1. What counts as a *significant* chance? This depends on various factors, and it may vary from society to society, from culture to culture. In general, the lower the degree of chance which counts as significant, the stronger the right to consent. And the stronger the right to consent, the greater the degree of freedom one has.
2. As we will see, this assumption is shared by the courts.

3. *8 Cal. 3rd,* p. 245 (This reference may appear mysterious to those not acquainted with the law. It is a reference to *California Reports,* a publication of the state of California.) My italics in the quotation.
4. He uses the term *self-determination* interchangeably with *self-decision.* See *8 Cal. 3rd*, pp. 242–243.
5. I assume that in practice we can usually tell when a person has enough information to make a rational choice. Theoretically, however, there are many problems here. To begin with, the word *rational* has many (related) meanings. We have indicated the meaning we intend here by a contrast between a *rational choice* and a *guess.* We all understand what someone means when he says, "I don't have enough information to make a rational choice; all I can do is guess." (It is easy to get confused here by the various meanings of *rational.* Because of these different meanings, it is true to say that it is rational to guess when you do not have enough information to make a rational choice. We must remember that the first occurrence of *rational* here cannot mean the same as its second occurrence. It cannot because in this second sense a rational choice is contrasted with a guess.)
6. Let us assume here that the parents have this right. We will discuss the role of parents in section 5.
7. *8 Cal. 3rd,* p. 244.
8. Ibid.
9. Ibid.
10. *8 Cal. 3rd,* p. 243. My italics in the quotation.
11. Our focus is exclusively on the contrast between free choice and the influence of other people. We are ignoring all other factors which influence choices.
12. There is an interesting—and, I think, accurate—description of how we weigh rights and desires at the beginning of Carl Jung's "On Psychic Energy," in *The Structure and Dynamics of the Psyche,* 2nd ed. (Princeton, N.J.: Princeton University Press, 1969), pp. 3–66.
13. This is one of the ways a right can be overridden. See Introduction, section 5.
14. Just how high a degree of probability is required? I do not think there is any definite degree we can state. The degree of probability which is appropriate will vary with the circumstances. Again, this calls for personal judgment.
15. We argued this point in Introduction, p. 15.
16. This case is reported in "The Adolescent Patient's Decision to Die," in Gorovitz, Andrew L. Jameton, John M. O'Connor, Eugene V. Perrin, Beverly Page St. Clair, Susan Sherwin (eds.), *Moral Problems in Medicine* (Englewood Cliffs, N.J.: Prentice-Hall, 1976), pp. 414–421.
17. See Ramsey, *The Patient as Person* (New Haven, Conn.: Yale University Press, 1972), p. 17.
18. Introduction, p. 15.
19. Carl Jung, *Mysterium Coniunctionis* 2nd ed. (Princeton, N.J.: Princeton University Press, 1970), p. 163.
20. Introduction, p. 12.
21. Introduction, p. 15.
22. Introduction, p. 12.

BIBLIOGRAPHY

Introductory

Brody, Howard. *Ethical Decisions in Medicine.* Boston: Little, Brown, 1976. Pp. 51–63.

Morris, Clarence. *Morris on Torts.* Brooklyn. Foundation Press, 1953. Pp. 27–35.

Ramsey, Paul. *The Patient as Person.* New Haven, Conn.: Yale University Press, 1972.

More Advanced

Fletcher, John. "Human Experimentation: Ethics in the Consent Situation." *Law and Contemporary Problems,* Vol. 32 (1967), p. 620.

Goldstein, Joseph. "For Harold Lasswell: Some Reflections on Human Dignity, Entrapment, Informed Consent and the Plea Bargain." *Yale Law Journal,* Vol. 84 (1973), p. 683.

Romano, J. "Reflections on Informed Consent." *Archives of General Psychiatry,* Vol. 32 (1974), p. 129.

Cobbs vs. *Grant. 8 Cal. 3rd* (1972), p. 229.

Hunter vs. *Brown. 484 P. 2nd* (1971), p. 1162.

Natanson vs. *Kline. 350 P. 2nd* (1960), p. 1093.

Slater vs. *Baker and Stapleton,* C.B. 95 *Eng. Rep.* 860 (1767).

TWO

Death, Dying, and Euthanasia: Dilemmas and Solutions

May life's sun upon thee smile,
Far from pain and far from sorrow.
Life is far too short, alas.
Death the kraken waits to drown you
in the sea of earth.

—The skolion of Seikilos

We identify with the power, energy, pleasure, and beauty of life, and in affirming life we tend to fear and resist death because we are afraid that death is the end of power, energy, pleasure, and beauty. But is affirming life always incompatible with accepting death? That is the central question of this chapter. The answer, I think, must be that affirming life is not always incompatible with accepting death. Consider, for example, what the composer Hector Berlioz writes in his memoirs about the death of his sister.

I have lost my eldest sister; she died of a cancer of the breast after six months of horrible suffering which drew heartrending screams from her day and night. My other sister who went to Grenoble to nurse her, and who did not leave her till the end, all but died from the fatigue and the painful impressions caused by this slow agony. And not a doctor dared to have the humanity to put an end to this martyrdom by making my sister inhale a bottle of chloroform. This is done to save a patient the pain of a surgical operation which lasts a quarter of a minute, and is not had recourse to in order to deliver one from a torture lasting six months. When it is proved certain that no remedy, nothing, not even time, can cure a dreadful disease; when death is evidently the supreme good, deliverance, joy, happiness! . . . The most horrible thing in the world for us living and sentient beings, is inexorable pain and suffering, pain without any possible compensation when it has reached this degree of intensity; and one must be barbarous, or stupid, or both at once, not to use the sure and easy means now at our disposal to bring it to an end. Savages are more intelligent and more humane.[1]

Berlioz is arguing for *euthanasia*—the inducing of a quiet and easy death. His point is that if we really affirm and value life, we should not

44

allow a person to linger on at the end of life in an agony that is pointless and dehumanizing. Does not the fact that we value life mean that
we should end life before it is debased by such gruesome and grotesque
suffering? Berlioz puts this question to us, and his own answer is clear:
Death is better than pointless suffering.

Is Berlioz right? We will consider this question in section 1. Whatever
our final answer, our attempt to answer it will raise other difficult
questions about euthanasia. When, if ever, should euthanasia be performed? What attitude should we have toward death? Is there a right
to die? And if there is, is suicide ever justified? Indeed, is there any
difference between suicide and euthanasia? Must a person always
consent to euthanasia? Or can someone else give proxy consent? These
last two questions are extremely important from a practical point of
view. But we must answer the others first in order to understand the
connection between euthanasia and consent.

1. Can death be better than life?

Berlioz makes a strong emotional plea for euthanasia. He is asking us
to imagine the suffering of his sister and to let ourselves feel the full
emotional impact of its horror. Once struck by the awfulness of her
pain, we would, Berlioz thinks, have to be "barbarous, or stupid, or
both at once" not to induce a quick, quiet, and easy death. In Berlioz's
eyes, to refuse to do this is to be less than human—"savages are more
intelligent and more humane."

Perhaps you find this emotional appeal moving. I certainly do. But
we should not let ourselves be convinced by an emotional plea which
does not also contain a well-reasoned argument. If we want to resolve
disagreements and controversies about euthanasia, we need to back up
our beliefs with good reasons. By explaining our reasons and by considering the reasons of others, we overcome the limits of our own
personal viewpoint and are able to reach agreement and resolve controversies. If, on the other hand, we let purely emotional appeals
convince us, we will remain confined within the boundaries of our
own limited point of view.

Now, the passage we quoted from Berlioz does contain an argument
in favor of euthanasia. The crucial claim on which this argument rests
is that his sister's suffering was pointless. According to Berlioz, she had
nothing to gain from living out her last six months in horrible pain.
If we agree with this claim, then we must also agree that his sister
should have been put to death in order to spare her the pain. Why?
Because it is true that when possible we should avoid pointless pain

and suffering.[2] But is his sister's pain really pointless? Different points of view lead to different answers to this question. The following examples illustrate several different points of view and answers.

Example 1. Mr. Lewis has cancer and is dying a slow and painful death. His pain is of the sort described in the following passage:

> Perhaps few persons who are not physicians can realize the influence which long-continued and unendurable pain may have upon the body and mind. The older books are full of cases in which after lancet wounds, the most terrible pain and local spasms resulted. When these lasted for weeks, the whole surface became hyperaesthetic, and the senses grew to be only avenues for fresh and increasing tortures, until every vibration, every change of light, and even . . . the effort to read brought on new agony. Under such torments the temper changes, the most amiable grow irritable, the soldier becomes a coward, the strongest man is scarcely less nervous than the most hysterical girl.[3]

Mr. Lewis's doctor is horrified by his patient's suffering and has given him a large supply of a powerful pain reliever. He warned Mr. Lewis that he should not take more than three pills every four hours, and that ten would be a fatal overdose. Despite this warning the doctor's intent was to provide Lewis with an easy means of suicide. Now, Lewis realizes and even appreciates his doctor's intent, but he nonetheless has his mind set against suicide. Lewis believes life is a gift from God, and that it is wrong for a person to refuse this gift by suicide or euthanasia. So he endures his intense and dehumanizing pain until the end.

Clearly, if we hold a religious view like this we will not think that the suffering of Berlioz's sister is pointless. On the contrary, her suffering is something she must endure if she is not to refuse the gift of life.

Example 2. Jean is a young woman of exceptional beauty who has a fatal disease. Her muscles will become progressively weaker until they are too weak to move her lungs. She faces a slow and agonizing death as she becomes progressively unable to breathe.[4] When Jean first learned of her disease, she made up her mind to die when her condition became so severe that she could not live a normal life. But when she reached that condition, she changed her mind and decided to live on as long as possible no matter what the cost. There was, she decided, always some slight chance that she would recover. Of course, a recovery would be a virtual miracle, but she decided she valued life so much that she wanted to live to the last possible moment hoping for a cure.

Again, if we share Jean's point of view, we will not think the suffering of Berlioz's sister is pointless. Rather, we will think the pain is something worth enduring in order to hold on to the slight hope of satisfying the desire for continued life. As the poet Julian Grenfell once wrote:

And life is color, warmth, and light,
And craving evermore for these . . .

Example 3. Kahn is a doctor who has discovered that he has cancer of the throat. The treatment for this is very painful and only delays death. It is not a cure. So, Kahn decides against treating his cancer. Instead, he plans to let the disease run its course until the pain becomes unbearable. At that point his plan is to kill himself. Kahn has no religious beliefs which prohibit this, and he can see no benefit to be derived from prolonging his suffering since—as a doctor—he is convinced there is no cure for his disease. The best course, he thinks, is to accept death when it is necessary to avoid intolerable pain and to live as well as he can until then.

Kahn's attitude is an old and respectable one. The ancient Roman philosopher Seneca, for example, held a similar attitude. According to Seneca

mere living is not a good, but living well. Accordingly the wise man will live as long as he ought, not as long as he can. . . . He always reflects concerning the quality, not the quantity, of his life. As soon as there are many events in his life that give him trouble and disturb his peace of mind, he sets himself free . . . he looks about carefully and sees whether he ought, or ought not, to end his life on that account. He holds that it makes no difference to him whether it comes later or earlier. He does not regard it with fear, as if it were a great loss; for no man can lose very much when but a driblet remains. It is not a question of dying earlier or later, but of dying well or ill. And dying well means escape from the danger of living ill.[5]

If this is our attitude toward death, we will certainly agree with Berlioz that his sister's suffering was pointless. In fact, this example shows us that Berlioz was right in thinking that affirming life and accepting death are compatible. We can consistently do both at once. Of course, there is still the question. Should we do both at once?

Whether we should depends on our attitude toward death. There are many possible attitudes to take—the three examples are hardly a complete list. So, it looks like each of us has only to figure out what his or her attitude toward death is in order to know what attitude to take toward euthanasia. But the situation is more complicated than that.

To begin with, most of us probably have more than one attitude toward death, and these attitudes are likely to be incompatible with each other. In one mood, you may think that what you would want to do when dying is stay alive as long as possible in hope of a miraculous cure. Yet in another frame of mind, you may decide that since death is inevitable it is pointless to endure terrible pain when dying. And so, you may come to the conclusion that you would commit suicide if you were experiencing unbearable pain. Of course, such conflicts involve other people as well. For example, suppose you are fatally ill and suffering a good deal of pain. You have decided you want to die before your pain becomes intolerable. But your doctor is very religious, and he refuses your request for euthanasia. He will not give you a fatal overdose of morphine, nor will he provide you with pills which you could use to commit suicide.

Such conflicts in ourselves and with others show that we must find answers to the following questions: What attitude should we take toward death? And, when the attitudes of different people conflict, how should this conflict be resolved? These are the questions we will consider in the next section.

2. Death, dying, and the right to die

What attitude should we take toward death? It is important to keep in mind that dying is something we do, and that we can do it badly or well. For example, one way for me to die badly would be to die in an intensive care unit. It is difficult to sleep in an intensive care unit since the lights are always on and since there is constant activity. Also, if one manages to fall asleep, one will probably be awakened in a few hours to take medication, or to have a blood sample drawn, or some such thing. Lack of sleep combined with the effects of painkilling drugs makes it difficult to think coherently. In addition, one may have a tube down one's throat which makes it impossible to talk and hence impossible to express those thoughts and desires one does have. I do not want to die like this. I would like to die with dignity, and lingering on in a semicoherent state in the intensive care unit does not fit my conception of a death with dignity.

But why should we care about how we die? The answer is straightforward: We should care because dying is our last chance for self-realization (in this life, at least). So, why not take advantage of it by dying well instead of badly? And, *dying well means dying in a way that promotes our self-realization.* Of course, this does not mean there is one right way to die. What promotes your self-realization may not promote mine. I do not want to die in an intensive care unit, but you might since it might best promote your self-realization to resist death in every possible way until the last possible moment.

Our attitude toward death, then, should be to view dying as an opportunity for self-realization, and therefore in deciding how to die we should determine which way of dying will be most conducive to our self-realization. However, as we have seen, your self-realization may be in conflict with another's. How are such conflicts to be resolved?

The central issue here is individual freedom: *We have the right to determine both how and when we will die.* This is so because to interfere with your decision about how or when to die is to interfere with your freedom and your right to self-determination. The right to die plays a central role in resolving conflicts about how to die. The best way to examine this role is to look at a number of different examples.

Case 1. Let us return to an example we considered at the end of section 1. You are fatally ill and in severe pain, and you have decided you want to die before the pain becomes intolerable. Your doctor, however, is very religious, and he refuses your request for euthanasia. He will not give you a fatal overdose of morphine, nor will he provide you with pills which you could use to commit suicide. How should this conflict be resolved?

You have the right to die—that is, the right to determine how and when to die. Of course, this does not mean you should automatically be allowed to carry out any decision you make about how and when you should die; there are circumstances in which your right to die can be justifiably overridden. But in this case we will assume there are no factors present which would justify overriding your right. Let us say that you are seventy-four years old, that you really are fatally ill, and that you have no responsibilities which you would be unjustifiably avoiding if your request for euthanasia were granted. In such a case you should be allowed to die, either by euthanasia or by suicide. What other answer can there be? After all, you have the right to die. So, respect for your freedom of choice demands that—in this case—you be allowed to die as you choose when you choose.

Your doctor thinks your decision is wrong, but that does not justify him in standing in your way. Unless we are justified in overriding it, a person's freedom must be respected. But this does not mean that your doctor must himself grant your request for euthanasia, for his own freedom to choose would be violated if he had to act against his own conscience. The most he need do is refer you to a doctor who is willing to perform euthanasia.

The legal status of euthanasia is unclear,[6] although some form of euthanasia is a common practice in most hospitals.[7] Our discussion so far shows that the legal status of euthanasia should be carefully examined since laws prohibiting euthanasia restrict freedom by overriding a person's right to die. But it is not obvious from what we have said so far that euthanasia should be legal.

The crucial question is: Can we write a law which allows euthanasia *and* which has adequate safeguards to protect people who do not want euthanasia? Safeguards are needed to protect patients who are not able to give or withhold free and informed consent to euthanasia: infants, children, people who are unconscious, senile, or mentally ill. Unless we can formulate adequate safeguards, it might be best to make euthanasia illegal. We will discuss this question more fully in section 6.

Case 2. Suppose I am a thirty-year-old man who is a professional skier. As a result of a racing accident I have lost a leg and an arm. Because of this I am extremely depressed, for my life was built around being a professional athlete. Now I am thinking of suicide. You visit me in my apartment and notice two large bottles of barbiturates in the medicine cabinet. You suspect—and you are right—that I obtained the drug in order to have a way of committing suicide. What should you do? Take the bottles away with you? Leave them but try to talk me out of suicide? Or say nothing about it at all?

I have the right to die. So, doesn't this mean you should not interfere? Shouldn't you leave the decision about suicide entirely up to me? No. It would be a mistake to think that the right to die means it would be wrong to interfere, for—in this case—there are considerations which override my right to die. To begin with, I am only thirty; I have at least half of my life ahead of me. And even without an arm and a leg I still have many possibilities for self-realization. Life as a professional skier is not the only life I can live. Also, we know that people generally recover from suicidal depressions like mine and begin a satisfying life again. These considerations argue strongly that you should do something about the possibility of my committing suicide. But what? Anything you do will be an infringement on my freedom. The question is how much of an infringement is justified? Should you confiscate the pills? Or should you leave the pills where they are and try to talk me out of suicide? You must use your own judgment. You should consider all the factors and make the best compromise you can between preventing my suicide and respecting my freedom. But no one can give you a rule for making such compromises.

It is worthwhile to consider the contrast between this example and the typical case of euthanasia. When someone requests euthanasia, he is (usually) dying. In addition, he has some reason to regard death and dying as positive. It is typically an escape from pain and also a final act of self-realization. So, euthanasia—or even suicide—at the end of life is a much different matter than the idea of suicide in this example which results from a severe but temporary depression in the middle of life. We can think of euthanasia as a form of suicide if we like, but we should not overlook these typical differences.

Case 3. This is an actual case:

> A seventy-nine-year-old man, languishing in a semicomatose condition in an acute care hospital, needed for survival an operation for renewal of a pacemaker. His wife, as guardian, refused permission for the surgery. The hospital then petitioned a court for appointment of a temporary guardian to authorize the surgery. A lower court judge in New York State complied and ordered performance of whatever procedures were necessary to "protect or sustain the health of life" of the patient. His wife lamented: "What has he got to live for? Nothing. He knows nothing, he has no memory whatsoever. He is turning into a vegetable. Isn't death better?"[8]

Who is right—the wife or the court? This question cannot be answered simply by appealing to the right to die. If the man were able to give or withhold free and informed consent, we could ask him how he wants to die. Since his death is clearly near, that is the key question; and if he gave us a free and informed answer, the right thing for us to do would be to respect his right to make that decision. But since he is "in a semi-comatose condition," he is not able to give or withhold consent, and that is what complicates matters. He cannot give or withhold consent to surgery; and, he cannot give or withhold consent to one or another way in which to die.

This is a situation involving proxy consent. The wife withholds consent to surgery on her husband's behalf, and in effect gives consent in his behalf to euthanasia—to letting him die. In doing so she comes into conflict with the hospital which takes legal measures to override her proxy consent. Now, in Chapter 1 we gave two principles, (P1) and (P2), which govern proxy consent.[9] If these principles are any good we should be able to use them to figure out what to do in cases like this one. And in fact we can use them in this way, but we are not ready to do so yet. We first need to return to the question: What attitude should we take toward death? In making a decision about whether another person should live or die we want to be sure we have a well-thought-out attitude toward death and dying.

3. Death, and life after death

To arrive at a well-thought-out attitude toward death, we have to consider the question of life after death. It is unusual to find such a discussion in modern, academic philosophy.[10] But the topic is extremely important. For one thing the question of survival after death arises for each of us, and we would like to know the answer. But more important, envisioning the possibility of an afterlife makes us confront the strength and power of our desire to survive death. We all have this desire, and it is essential that we acknowledge its force and find some way to deal with it. Dealing with the desire to survive death does not seem so important when we are young, for then we are shaping our future and are deeply involved in plans that hold before us the pleasant prospect of future satisfaction and fulfillment. But life leads to death, and the farther along we are in life the more difficult it is to ignore the fact that death is approaching.

It is difficult to ignore the approach of death, but the strength of our desire for life makes it equally difficult to accept it. Carl Jung says that

> ordinarily we cling to our past and remain stuck in the illusion of youthfulness. Being old is highly unpopular. Nobody seems to consider that not being able to grow old is just as absurd as not being able to outgrow child's-size shoes. A still infantile man of thirty is surely to be deplored, but a youthful septuagenarian—isn't that delightful? And yet both are perverse, lacking in style, psychological monstrosities. A young man who does not fight and conquer has missed the best part of his youth, and an old man who does not know how to listen to the secrets of the brooks, as they tumble down from the peaks, makes no sense; he is a spiritual mummy who is nothing but a rigid relic of the past. He stands apart from life, mechanically repeating himself to the last triviality.[11]

Jung's point is that the conflict between the desire for life and the awareness of death's approach can destroy the energy and vitality of a person's life and reduce him to "a spiritual mummy who is nothing but a rigid relic of the past." We will not resolve this conflict by ignoring it. The paradox of maturity is that we remain vitally alive only by accepting and preparing for death.

But how are we to prepare for it? There is no general answer. Each person must find the answer that fits him or her as an individual—the answer that best promotes self-realization. The one general truth we can state is that it is a bad idea to deny death, to refuse to accept it. This truth has practical consequences for the treatment of dying patients.

Doctors often think it is part of their duty as physicians to maintain life for as long as possible. Consciously or unconsciously, they regard themselves as fighting a war against death, and they will allow neither peace nor compromise with the enemy. Such an attitude conflicts with the idea that a person should accept death and prepare for it. If this is true, then a doctor should not think it is in all circumstances part of his duty to his patient to maintain life for as long as possible. Rather, when a patient is clearly dying, his doctor should try to find out how the patient thinks of death and help him accept and prepare for it.

It is worthwhile to digress briefly and discuss the question of whether or not we really do survive death. It is often difficult for people to approach this question with an open mind. Those who have strong religious beliefs tend to insist that we survive death. Those who are not religious tend to regard belief in an afterlife as a superstition which is unworthy of an educated and sophisticated mind. But the fact is there is some evidence that we do survive death. We need to evaluate this evidence and determine how we should let it affect our attitude toward death. There are three sources of evidence, and we will consider them in turn.

Reports from people who have "died". The first source of evidence is a product of modern medical science. Modern medical techniques make it possible to revive people who have "died." Here is a typical example. A patient begins to have a severe heart attack. As the team of doctors rush in to help, his heart stops, he stops breathing, and he shows no signs of life. The doctors, however, succeed in reviving the patient. Let us call this a near-death episode. The patient does not die, but before he is revived he shows all the clinical signs of death.

Patients who have had near-death episodes sometimes report that they had certain experiences while "dead." One remarkable and important fact about these reports is that they all describe very similar experiences. This fact caught the attention of Dr. Raymond Moody several years ago. Since then he has extensively interviewed patients who have had near-death episodes, and he has put together the following summary of what people say happens to them, which captures all the common elements reported.

A man is dying and, as he reaches the point of greatest physical distress, he hears himself pronounced dead by his doctor. He begins to hear an uncomfortable noise, a loud ringing or buzzing, and at the same time feels himself moving very rapidly through a long tunnel. After this, he suddenly finds himself outside of his own physical body, but still in the immediate physical environment, and he sees his own body from a distance, as though he is a spectator. He watches the resuscitation attempt from this unusual vantage point and is in a state of emotional upheaval.

After a while, he collects himself and becomes more accustomed to his odd condition. He notices that he still has a "body," but one of a very different nature and with very different powers from the physical body he has left behind. Soon other things begin to happen. Others come to meet and to help him. He glimpses the spirits of relatives and friends who have already died, and a loving, warm spirit of a kind he has never encountered before—a being of light—appears before him. This being asks him a question, nonverbally, to make him evaluate his life and helps him along by showing him a panoramic, instantaneous playback of the major events of his life. At some point he finds himself approaching some sort of barrier or border, apparently representing the limit between earthly life and the next life. Yet, he finds that he must go back to the earth, that the time for his death has not yet come. At this point he resists, for by now he is taken up with his experiences in the afterlife and does not want to return. He is overwhelmed by intense feelings of joy, love, and peace. Despite his attitude, though, he somehow reunites with his physical body and lives.

Later he tries to tell others, but he has trouble doing so. In the first place, he can find no human words adequate to describe these unearthly episodes. He also finds that others scoff, so he stops telling other people. Still, the experience affects his life profoundly, especially his views about death and its relationship to life.[12]

What are we to make of the fact that a very large number of people have reported these experiences? Clearly, one explanation is that we really do survive death (at least for a while). But another explanation is possible: it might be that the experiences reported were just hallucinations, produced perhaps by abnormal brain activity. But the hallucination explanation faces two stumbling blocks. First, if we are dealing with hallucinations, why do people always "hallucinate" the same things? Wouldn't hallucinations show more individual variation? Second, the reports people give frequently contain accurate descriptions of what their doctors did when attempting to revive them. "He watches the resuscitation attempt from this unusual vantage point. . . ." In his book, *Lectures on Psychical Research,* the philosopher C. D. Broad describes several cases in which a person who was "dead" or near death seemed to "leave his body" and obtain accurate knowledge of events which occurred while he was unconscious.[13] Patients were frequently able to describe accurately what was done and said while they were being revived. The were also able to describe the nurses and doctors who revived them but whom they had never before seen. It is difficult to see how the hallucination explanation can account for these facts.

Historical reports. The case against the hallucination explanation becomes stronger when we consider the second source of evidence for survival after death: historical reports of "out of the body" experiences. Although it is only recently that such reports have become well-known, they have been given since the earliest times.[14] There is a striking feature of these reports. The experiences they describe are all more or less like the composite description quoted from Moody. This casts more doubt on the hallucination explanation. Are we to believe that people from different times and different cultures "hallucinated" basically the same events as the twentieth-century Americans interviewed by Dr. Moody?

Religious traditions. Religions provide us with our final source of evidence. Almost all religions tell us that we survive death. The Tibetan *Book of the Dead,* for example, contains explicit instructions about how to conduct yourself in the transition between this life and the next (instructions that bear remarkable similarities to the reports collected by Moody). There is a tendency to push religious writings like this aside as products of a superstitious and unscientific age. But, given the above facts, perhaps we should take them more seriously. Certainly the fact that the religious tradition of survival agrees with recent medical investigations should not be ignored. It is important that approaches from both the religious and scientific point of view support the idea that we continue to live after death.

Such is the evidence. How should we let it affect our attitude toward death? Should we believe in an afterlife or not? Many find it unreasonable to accept survival after death on the basis of the above evidence.[15] The reason for this is that the idea of an afterlife conflicts with other basic beliefs many of us hold; in particular, that the mind is just a product of brain activity, that everything mental results from electrochemical activity in a physical nervous system, and that when this activity ceases, all mental activity ceases. This is a scientific hypothesis which may or may not turn out to be correct. I certainly do not think that the evidence for an afterlife we have cited is strong enough to overturn this hypothesis. Still, it would be unreasonable to ignore or deny the evidence.

So, the best attitude on the question of life after death is to keep an open mind until the conflict is resolved. An open mind is also useful in accepting and preparing for death because it counteracts our tendency to regard death as completely negative, as the absolute end of life.

4. Death and the doctor's role

We have seen that a well-thought-out attitude toward death—one in which we accept death and prepare for it—should be the basis for deciding whether another person should live or die—cases involving proxy consent to euthanasia.

At the end of Section 2 we gave an example which involved the issue of proxy consent to euthanasia, but we did not answer the questions which it raised. Let us return to that example now. Recall that we were considering a seventy-nine-year-old man who was in a semicomatose state. He needed an operation to renew his pacemaker; otherwise, he was going to die. His wife refused to consent to the surgery, but

> the hospital then petitioned a court for appointment of a temporary guardian to authorize surgery. A lower court judge in New York State complied and ordered performance of whatever procedures were necessary to "protect or sustain the health or life" of the patient. His wife lamented: "What has he got to live for? Nothing. He knows nothing, he has no memory whatsoever. He is turning into a vegetable. Isn't death better?"

The unanswered question was: Who is right—the wife, or the court? A good way to approach a question like this is think up the strongest case you can for each side and then compare the cases to see which is stronger. In this way we force ourselves to look at the issue from both points of view, a good idea if we want to make a reasonable and fair decision.

The wife's case. The wife insists that performing the surgery will not serve any useful purpose ("He is turning into a vegetable. Isn't death better?"), and this is a point with which we must agree; that is, we must agree with it given that we think the most sensible approach to death is to accept and prepare for it. The court's order is incompatible with this approach, for the court ordered the doctors to "protect or sustain the health or life of the patient." But we have argued that it should not always be part of the doctor's role to maintain life. On the contrary, when a patient is clearly dying his doctor should help the patient accept death and prepare for it. Of course, a doctor must respect his patient's rights. If his patient wants to use every possible means to extend and maintain life, that is within his rights, and his doctor obviously cannot justify forcing death on him. But, equally, when a patient is dying and accepts it a doctor should not think it is still part of his duty or role as a doctor to maintain the patient's life.

In the case before us the man is clearly dying—slowly. The person who knows him best—his wife—has decided that death is better for him. So, why should life be forced on the old man? How can the court justify its decision? They might claim that a doctor is responsible for the life of his patient and must always maintain and protect that life. But we have seen this is not always so.

In defense of the court. The court can defend itself by pointing out that we have overlooked an essential point. This is: The man himself does not give consent to his death. His wife is the one who does. By withholding consent to surgery she in effect consents to euthanasia, to letting her husband die. Now, the court could claim that in cases where the patient himself accepts death and consents to it, the doctor is no longer responsible for the patient's life. But when the patient is unable to give consent the doctor must—the court could say—maintain the patient's life. Wouldn't any other course run the risk of interfering in the most drastic way with the patient's right to self-determination by causing his death?

A comparison of the cases. There is some truth in what the wife says, and there is some truth in the court's defense. But both perspectives are too simplified to be correct. To see what is right and wrong in each, we have to realize that the question of proxy consent to euthanasia arises in two quite different situations. In one situation there is someone—like the man's wife—who knows what the patient's attitude toward euthanasia is. In the other situation there is no one who knows what the patient's attitude is.

As an example of the first sort of situation, suppose the seventy-nine-year-old man's wife knew that her husband himself thought that death would be better for him. We can imagine that they had discussed death many times, and that her husband had clearly and repeatedly expressed his desire to die rather than linger on as a vegetable. In this sort of case the wife is right and the court is wrong. This is clear if we recall (P1), one of our two principles about proxy consent.[16]

(P1) applies in those cases in which someone is available who can figure out what the patient would consent to if he were capable of giving consent. (P1) says:

A person x ought to give consent to an action A on behalf of another person y if and only if x has good reason to think that y would give free and informed consent to A if y were able to give free and informed consent.

In our present case x is the wife, y is the husband, and the action A is euthanasia—letting the husband die by refusing surgery. The wife knows her husband would consent to dying, so she is right to refuse surgery and opt for death. According to (P1) it is right for her to make this choice on her husband's behalf.[17] Given this choice the doctor is relieved of his responsibility for the patient's life. It is no longer part of his responsibility to maintain that life. If he did try to maintain the man's life, he would be interfering with his right to consent.

The situation is much different, however, if we turn to cases in which there is no one present who knows what the patient's attitude toward euthanasia is. Suppose, for example, that the seventy-nine-year-old man does not have a wife. Suppose that, like many very old people, he lives alone without family or friends. Since he is only semiconscious he cannot give or withhold free and informed consent to surgery, and he cannot express his wishes about how he would like to die. This is a case in which our other principle about proxy consent, (P2), applies.[18] To state (P2), let x be the doctor and y, the seventy-nine-year-old man. Then, (P2) says:

With respect to y, x should perform those therapeutic actions—and *only* those therapeutic actions—which are necessary to maintain y's physical and mental health.

Now, given (P2) it looks like this time the court is right. (P2) says the doctor should perform those actions necessary to maintain the physical and mental health of the patient. Doesn't this mean the doctor should keep the man alive?

No, it does not. It only means the doctor must not kill the old man. To this extent we can agree with the court. But the doctor may let the man die. To see that this is true, we first have to convince ourselves that there really is a morally important distinction between *killing* and *letting die*. Once this distinction is clear we can return to the case of the seventy-nine-year-old man.

5. Killing and letting die

We can see the distinction between killing and letting die from the following example. Suppose three men are sailing in the ocean when their boat strikes an underwater reef and begins to sink. Two of the three are knocked unconscious by the collision, and the one who is still conscious realizes he can save only one of the two unconscious men. Both men are his good friends, and he does not know how to choose between them. But one man seems to be less badly hurt, so he pulls him up on the sinking boat and begins to swim ashore with the other. He hopes the friend he left on the boat will regain consciousness in time to save himself, but he doubts it since the boat is sinking fast. Unfortunately, the man does not gain consciousness and drowns.

Did the man who was conscious kill the friend he left on the boat? Most of us will answer *no*. If we do use the word *kill* to describe this situation we run the risk of overlooking an important distinction between this case and clear cases of killing. Think about what happens in clear cases of killing. Somebody—the killer—performs an action—say, shooting a gun—which causes another person's death. And the killer performed this action because he wanted it to result in that person's death. Now, in our example the conscious man did not pull his friend onto the sinking boat because he wanted to cause his friend's death. His purpose was exactly the opposite: He hoped he would regain consciousness and save himself.

For the sake of clarity it is best to restrict the word *kill* to cases in which a person does something because he wants to cause another person's death. So, we will not say that the conscious man killed his friend. But he did let him die. The difference between killing and letting die lies in the reason for the action. When we let someone die we act in a way that results in his death. In addition, we believe at the time of our action that it will probably cause the person's death. But we do not perform the action *because* we want the person to die. We have some other reason—like the conscious man in the boating disaster. His reason for abandoning his friend was to save the life of the other man. He knew he could not rescue both of them. He let one friend die, as it turned out, but he did not kill him.

So, there is a genuine distinction between killing and letting die. This distinction is important because it helps resolve questions about proxy consent to euthanasia. To see this, let us return once more to the case of the seventy-nine-year-old man.

Remember, we are supposing the man lives alone, has no wife, and no other available family or friends. He needs surgery to live, but he cannot give or withhold free and informed consent to surgery because he is only semiconscious. In the last section we saw that (P2) applies here. According to it the doctor should perform those actions—and only those actions—which maintain the physical and mental health of the man.

This means the doctor should not kill the man. To state the obvious, killing—causing death because you want to cause death—is not an action which maintains health. In cases like this, in which (P2) applies, killing is ruled out.[19] Killing ought to be considered only in those cases in which the patient himself is able to give consent, or in which someone else who knows the patient's attitude toward euthanasia is able to give proxy consent (where (P1) applies).

But killing is one thing and letting die is another, and we claimed that it was permissible for the doctor to let the man die. In fact, we can make a stronger claim: (P2) *requires* that the doctor let the man die. Recall exactly what (P2) says about this case: the doctor should perform those actions—*and only those actions*—which maintain the physical and mental health of the old man. The crucial question is: Which actions maintain health? Certainly, making the man comfortable and reducing his pain count as such actions. But does surgery to renew his pacemaker count? I do not think so. The man is degenerating into a vegetable-like state. Surgery will not stop this process; it will just prolong it by keeping the man's body functioning while he continues to degenerate. Is this maintaining health? To see that the answer to this question should be *no,* we need to explain the concept of health.

6. Two concepts of health

Actually, there are two different but related concepts of health. We will call one concept *biological health* and the other *overall health.* The easiest way to explain the distinction between them is to sketch an account of each.

To see what biological health is, think of the body and mind as a complex system. This system functions typically in certain specific ways that are conducive to continued existence of the organism and also to reproduction. We will not try to say what these "specific ways" are. This is a task for medicine and the appropriate medically related sciences. All we need to note is that *there are* certain specific ways in which the body and mind function. When a subsystem is functioning in the specific ways which are typical of it, we will say it is functioning normally. For example, the lungs function to extract carbon dioxide from the blood and replace it with oxygen, and we could explain how this exchange of oxygen for carbon dioxide is necessary if life is to continue from moment to moment. The lungs illustrate a bodily function. But we could also explain how a mental capacity like thinking contributes to survival and reproduction since the ability to think is certainly necessary to dealing in an effective way with our environment.

Roughly speaking, a person is biologically healthy provided that his body and mind are functioning in those typical ways which are conducive to his continued existence and to his ability to reproduce—in other words, provided his mind and body are functioning normally.[20] Now, the old man in the pacemaker example is certainly not biologically healthy, for his heart and brain are not functioning normally. Still, surgery to renew his pacemaker would certainly help maintain his biological health since it would help his heart to function in a way much closer to normal. So, if we understood the word *health* in (P2) as meaning biological health, (P2) would actually require that we perform the surgery.

But should we understand the word *health* in (P2) as meaning biological health? I do not think so. Instead, we should understand it to mean overall health. The best way to see what overall health is, is to ask: Why do we care about being biologically healthy? What reason do we have for staying alive and reproducing? We saw in the Introduction that we have two reasons. First, we have a personal reason for staying alive, and that is to pursue our self-realization. Second, we also have a nonpersonal reason for living—namely, to maximize self-realization in general. This is also a reason for reproducing since one way to maximize self-realization is to ensure the continued existence of our species since we are a species capable of experiencing self-realization.

We should care about biological health because some degree of biological health is needed for the effective pursuit of self-realization, and when we are unable to pursue self-realization, biological health loses its point. So, when we are trying to "stay healthy," it is not just biological health we should aim at, but that degree of biological health which will allow us to pursue self-realization effectively.

We can distinguish between biological health and overall health by defining overall health this way: *a person is healthy overall provided that he is biologically healthy to a degree that allows him to pursue self-realization effectively.* The point of this distinction between biological health and overall health is that you can be biologically healthy without being healthy overall.

In the case of the old man who is degenerating it still would be possible to maintain his biological health by renewing his pacemaker. This would ensure his continued physical functioning. But continued physical functioning would not maintain the old man's overall health. He has, in fact, lost his overall health because he has lost the capacity for self-realization. What is the point of maintaining biological health in this case? The answer must be: no point. Biological health has a point to it only insofar as it is conducive to self-realization. Biological health is important because overall health is important. When we lose our overall health by losing our capacity for self-realization, biological health ceases to be important. It makes sense, then, to understand the word *health* in (P2) to mean overall health. It is overall health that we care about. So, from now on this is how we will interpret (P2). And with (P2) interpreted this way, it requires that we let the old man die.

We can summarize the results of our discussion of killing and letting die and of health by distinguishing between *active* and *passive* euthanasia. Active euthanasia is killing the patient. Passive euthanasia consists in letting the patient die. Active euthanasia always requires consent. Either the patient himself must consent, or someone who knows the patient's attitude toward euthanasia must consent on his behalf. Passive euthanasia does not always require the patient's consent. Of course, if the patient is able to give or withhold free and informed consent to either form of euthanasia, then his consent must be obtained. However, if we are in a case in which (P2) applies, consent to letting die is not necessary. The crucial question is what maintains health.

7. Conclusion

We have argued that various forms of euthanasia are morally permissible, but are they legal? Let us consider active euthanasia first. Active euthanasia certainly looks like murder, which is of course illegal. The fact that a patient consents to active euthanasia is not a legal defense to the charge of murder; that is the current law.[21] This law should be changed. In those cases in which active euthanasia is morally permissible, it should also be legal. Why should our laws force us to act contrary to what is moral? There is only one possible justification for such a situation; namely, that we cannot write a law which allows active euthanasia and which has adequate safeguards. We need safeguards to protect patients who are incapable of giving free and informed consent to euthanasia: infants, children, people who are unconscious, senile, or mentally ill. I think such a law can be written; in fact, (P1) and (P2) show us basically how to do it. We should require in such cases that a person who knows the patient's attitude toward euthanasia give or withhold consent on behalf of the patient. Of course, adequate measures must be taken to ensure that the person giving proxy consent does know the patient well enough, and that he or she will sincerely attempt to act in accord with (P1). If no such person is available, (P2) applies. In these cases only passive euthanasia should be legal, and it should be legal only when it can be clearly shown that those medical procedures which would keep the patient alive do not do anything to maintain his health.

The legal situation with respect to passive euthanasia is unclear. In America no doctor has been brought to trial for passive euthanasia.[22] In addition, California has recently passed a right-to-die bill.[23] Basically, this bill makes passive euthanasia legal in certain circumstances. Roughly, you can specify—in a document called a *living will*—whether or not you want passive euthanasia if you are unconscious and dying. A living will, if properly made in sound mind, is legally binding on the doctor. The position of the right-to-die bill agrees partly with what we have said about the right to die. It states:

> The Legislature finds that adult persons have the fundamental right to control the decisions relating to the rendering of their own medical care, including the decision to have life-sustaining procedures withheld or withdrawn in instances of a terminal condition.
>
> The Legislature further finds that modern medical technology has made possible the artificial prolongation of human life beyond natural limits.
>
> The Legislature further finds that, in the interest of protecting individual autonomy, such prolongation of life for persons with a terminal condition may cause loss of patient dignity and unnecessary pain and suffering, while providing nothing medically necessary or beneficial to the patient.[24]

The bill says that the right to die may justifiably be exercised when a person is in a "terminal condition" for which nothing "medically beneficial can be done." The bill allows passive euthanasia only given the patient's prior consent as spelled out in writing beforehand. We have argued, on the contrary, that passive euthanasia does not always require consent.

THEORETICAL FOUNDATIONS

We have left one important theoretical question unanswered: *Why* do we have the right to determine how and when we should die? According to our definition of what a right is,[25] you have the right to determine how and when you should die provided that (a) there is a reason why others should not interfere with how and when you choose to die, (b) each person has this reason simply and solely by virtue of being a person. Therefore, to show that you have the right to die, we must show that (a) and (b) are true.

To do this we need to take note of certain facts about death. To begin with we should remind ourselves that death is the end of consciousness (in this life, at least). As such, it is our last chance for self-realization. Since death is inevitable, this last chance is forced on each of us. It makes sense to make the best possible use of this last chance, and so each of us has a reason to die well, to die in a way that promotes self-realization. Now, since we have a reason not to interfere with a person's pursuit of self-realization, it follows that we have a reason not to interfere with a person's decision about how and when he or she should die.

We have reached this conclusion by appealing to facts which are true of people simply and solely by virtue of their being persons. So, (a) and (b) are true. There is a reason why others should not interfere with your decision about how and when to die, and each person has this reason simply and solely by virtue of being a person. Therefore, you do have the right to die.

FURTHER QUESTIONS

1. In section 1, we illustrated three attitudes toward death. What other typical attitudes are there?

2. Is suicide sometimes justified? If so, when?

3. Given that we always value life to some extent, isn't death always to that same extent an evil?

4. Suppose the doctor in the case of the seventy-nine-year-old man did not perform surgery *both* because he thought it would not maintain his health, *and* because he wanted the old man to die (thought he would be better off dead). Would his not performing surgery be morally justifiable?

NOTES

1. Quoted in Stanley Reiser, "The Dilemma of Euthanasia in Modern Medical History," in John A. Behnke and Sissela Bok (eds.), *The Dilemmas of Euthanasia* (New York: Anchor/Doubleday, 1975), pp. 27–49. The quotation occurs in pp. 27–28.
2. Introduction, p. 15.
3. S. W. Mitchel, *Injuries to the Nerves and Their Consequences* (Philadelphia: Lippincott, 1872).
4. Amyotrophic lateral sclerosis is such a disease.
5. Seneca, *Epistula Morales,* "On Suicide," reprinted in Samuel Gorovitz, Andrew L. Jameton, John M. O'Connor, Eugene V. Perrin, Beverly Page St. Clair, Susan Sherwin (eds.), *Moral Problems in Medicine* (Englewood Cliffs, N.J.: Prentice-Hall, 1976), p. 376.
6. See the following two essays in John A. Behnke and Sissela Bok (eds.), *The Dilemmas of Euthanasia* (New York: Anchor/Doubleday, 1975): David W. Meyers, "The Legal Aspects of Voluntary Medical Euthanasia," pp. 51–68; Norman L. Cantor, "Law and the Termination of an Incompetent Patient's Life-preserving Care," pp. 69–106.
7. It is common in the sense that hospitals classify certain patients as "no code." This means that after a heart attack (for example) no attempt to revive the patient will be made. They will simply let the patient die if he cannot recover on his own.
8. *The New York Times,* January 29, 1972, p. 42. This case is quoted and discussed in the essay by Cantor cited in note 6.
9. Chapter 1, pp. 28–35.
10. There are notable exceptions. For example, C. D. Broad discusses the arguments for survival in his major work on the philosophy of mind, *The Mind and Its Place in Nature* (London: Routledge & Kegan Paul, 1925), Chaps. 11 and 12.
11. Carl Jung, "The Soul and Death," in *The Structure and Dynamics of the Psyche* (Princeton, N.J.: Princeton University Press, 1969), p. 407.
12. Raymond A. Moody, *Life After Life* (New York: Bantam, 1976), pp. 121–123.
13. C. D. Broad, *Lectures on Psychical Research* (London: Routledge & Kegan Paul, 1962), Chap. 7.
14. See Moody, *Life After Life,* pp. 109–128.
15. See Moody, *Life After Life,* pp. 155–177.
16. Chapter 1, p. 34.
17. Assuming that no circumstances justify overriding her husband's right to consent.
18. Chapter 1, p. 35.
19. Unless, of course, there are very exceptional circumstances which justify the killing. The statement that killing is ruled out is meant to apply to the typical situations we most often encounter.
20. This holds only "roughly speaking" because it is not true that every deviation

from normal functioning makes you *un*healthy. For example, a person who has double-jointed fingers is not unhealthy even though his fingers do not function normally. A deviation makes you biologically unhealthy if and only if it reduces your chances for continued existence and reproduction. We can take this as a definition of being biologically *un*healthy and then define biological health as *not* being biologically unhealthy.

21. See, for example, the discussion at the beginning of David W. Meyers, "The Legal Aspects of Voluntary Medical Euthanasia," in John A. Behnke and Sissela Bok (eds.), *The Dilemmas of Euthanasia* (New York: Anchor/Doubleday, 1975), pp. 51–68.

22. This is reported in Norman L. Cantor, "Law and the Termination of an Incompetent Patient's Life-preserving Care," in John A. Behnke and Sissela Bok, *The Dilemmas of Euthanasia* (Anchor/Doubleday, 1975), pp. 69–106.

23. California Assembly Bill, No. 3060; this bill went into effect January 1, 1977.

24. Ibid., p. 2.

25. Introduction, p. 12.

BIBLIOGRAPHY

Introductory

Behnke, John A. and **Bok, Sissela** eds. *The Dilemmas of Euthanasia.* New York: Anchor/Doubleday, 1975.

More Advanced

Broad, C. D. *The Mind and Its Place in Nature.* London: Routledge & Kegan Paul, 1925. Chaps. 11 and 12.

Dinello, Daniel. "On Killing and Letting Die," in Samuel Gorovitz, et al. (eds.) *Moral Problems in Medicine.* Englewood Cliffs, N.J.: Prentice-Hall, 1976. Pp. 281–283.

Jung, Carl. "The Soul and Death." In *The Structure and Dynamics of the Psyche.* Princeton, N.J.: Princeton University Press, 1969.

Moody, Raymond A. *Life After Life.* New York: Bantam, 1976.

Moody, Raymond A. *Reflections on Life After Life.* New York: Bantam, 1977.

THREE

The Problem of Abortion and Infanticide

Suppose you and your husband both thought you wanted a child, and so you became pregnant. But now the daily fact of pregnancy has made you reconsider the whole question of having children, and you have both decided that you are not ready to raise a child. Should you have an abortion? Or is it wrong to kill the developing fetus simply because you do not feel ready to raise the child it will become? Here is another situation. Suppose you really do want a child, but suppose also that the child you bear has a birth defect which will make it severely handicapped and mentally retarded. Do you have to raise it? Or is infanticide morally permissible here? Can you let the child die? Or even kill it?

Abortion is common and infanticide—in the form of passive euthanasia, letting die—is more widespread than most people realize. It is estimated that sixty out of every thousand newborn infants will need some form of intensive care.[1] In certain cases it is not uncommon to withhold the needed treatment and let the infant die. For example, this might be done if the infant is missing part of its brain (if it is anencephalic). From a purely practical point of view, then, it is important to discuss abortion and infanticide in some detail. We should determine whether practices which are common are morally justifiable.

1. The case against abortion

Suppose that Karen, an eighteen-year-old college freshman, is raped walking back from the library to her dorm. As a result Karen becomes pregnant. She absolutely does not want to have the child and wants an abortion. Her father, who has very strict religious views, tries to convince her that abortion is always wrong no matter what the circumstances. He also refuses to pay for the abortion. Karen, however, does not see why she should have to bear the child of the man who raped her, and so she arranges for the abortion without her father's knowledge or assistance.

Who is right—Karen or her father? Is abortion always wrong? Or is it permissible in certain circumstances? In particular, is it permissible in Karen's case? Probably most of us would agree that abortion is permissible in rape cases like Karen's. But it is still important to find reasons which back up this view. If we want to understand our moral views, and if we want to know what to say about abortion in unclear cases, we need reasons. To find them we will give two arguments—one for and one against abortion. The antiabortion argument tries to show that abortion is always wrong. This extreme position rests on two assumptions. The proabortion argument rejects these assumptions and holds that abortion is morally permissible in the case of Karen as well as in certain other cases.

Most people who oppose abortion do so because they think the developing fetus is a person. The usual argument offered in support of this idea begins by asking us to consider the sequence of development from the moment of conception to early childhood. When we do this, what we see is a continuous, unbroken line of growth and change. There are no breaks or gaps in this line which we can point to as definitely marking the change from being a nonperson to being a person. Of course, we could impose an arbitrary division on this smooth line of development and simply stipulate that before a given point—for example, the tenth week of pregnancy—the fetus is not a person, but that after that point it is a person. But opponents of abortion often claim any stipulation like this is so arbitrary that it cannot be justified. And they conclude from this that *we ought to regard a fetus as a person from even the moment of conception.* This is the first assumption. We will object to it later in section 3. Right now our question is: Granting the assumption, can we ever justify abortion? Since we are presenting the antiabortion view first, we want to find the strongest possible argument for a *no* answer to this question.

The strongest argument I know is based on an appeal to the right to consent. Since we are assuming that the fetus is a person, we must agree that it has the right to give or withhold free and informed consent to medical procedures performed on it—in particular, to abortion. Of course, we cannot possibly ask the fetus if it consents, and it is exactly this impossibility which is the key point in the antiabortion argument. Since we cannot ask the fetus what it wants, we must have someone else give or withhold proxy consent on behalf of the fetus.[2] From the antiabortion point of view, it does not matter who gives or withholds proxy consent in this situation as consent should always be withheld. Why? Because—so the antiabortion argument claims—the principles which apply to proxy consent establish that consent should always be withheld in such cases.

We must ask whether the principles which govern proxy consent, (P1) and (P2),[3] really have the consequence that abortion is always wrong. To answer this question suppose that, in the case of Karen, you are the one who represents the fetus in the decision about abortion. You are to give or withhold consent on behalf of the fetus. The principles (P1) and (P2) are intended to guide you in making such a decision. Now, to apply these principles you first have to determine whether there are any circumstances which justify overriding the fetus' right to consent. The reason is that neither (P1) nor (P2) apply if such circumstances exist; they simply are not intended to deal with such cases. *It is a crucial assumption of the antiabortion argument that no circumstances ever justify overriding the fetus' right to give or withhold consent to abortion.* This is the second assumption, which we will argue against in section 5. For now let us grant it and see what follows.

Once we grant the assumption, what follows is that you should make your decision in accord with either (P1) or (P2). But which principle should you use?

Suppose you try to use (P1). Then you have to know certain facts about the fetus. To see what these facts are, consider what (P1) says when applied to this case:

> You ought to give consent to abortion on behalf of the fetus if and only if you have good reason to think the fetus would consent to the abortion if it were capable of giving free and informed consent.

So, to apply (P1) you need to know that the fetus would consent to its own abortion. Can you know this? I do not see how. A fetus has no conceptions of life, death, health, illness, pain, and suffering.[4] How, then, could it possibly make choices which involve these concepts? Of course, we can imagine the child it will develop into making all sorts of choices. But to do this is not to imagine the fetus making choices. So, there is simply no answer to the question of what the fetus would choose if it could give or withhold consent.

This means that (P1) does not apply. But when (P1) does not apply, (P2) does, for (P2) covers just those cases in which we cannot figure out what the person would choose. Applied to this case (P2) says:

> With respect to the fetus, you should perform those therapeutic actions—and only those therapeutic actions—which maintain the physical and mental health of the fetus.

Does an abortion maintain the health of the fetus? Surely it does not. Abortion means death, for most abortions are performed so early in pregnancy that there is no chance of keeping the fetus alive. And, even in late abortions where this might be possible, the fetus is allowed to die. The death of the fetus is usually part of the reason for the abortion.

Generally, people opt for abortion because—for one or another reason—they do not want the child.

Since abortion does not maintain the health of the fetus, you must withhold consent. This is what (P2) says when applied to this case. Now, given the assumption that no circumstances justify overriding the fetus' right to consent, this means that the abortion should not be performed. Abortion—according to the antiabortion argument—is morally unjustifiable in the case of Karen; and, in fact, it is unjustifiable in *every* case, for the antiabortion argument is completely general and can be applied to every case in which the question of abortion arises.

The antiabortion argument must be wrong. If we accepted it we would have to oppose abortion even when it was necessary to save the woman's life. We would also have to believe that women who, like Karen, were pregnant as the result of a rape had to bear the child of the man who raped them. I find these conclusions appalling and cannot believe them, and I think we can find good reasons to support this emotional reaction and show that it is morally right. To do this we need to show that the antiabortion argument rests on false assumptions. There are just two assumptions to question. One is the assumption that a fetus is a person; the other, that no circumstances ever override the fetus' right to consent (a right it has on the assumption that it is a person).

2. What is a person?

The antiabortion argument assumes that a fetus is a person, but it does not tell us what a person is. If we ask: What is a person? different people will give us different answers. The religiously minded may tell us that a person consists of a body and a soul combined, and so, on this view, a fetus will count as a person provided a soul has combined with its body. Others will offer a completely nonreligious account of what a person is. Now, different accounts of what a person is lead to different answers to the question of whether a fetus is a person. On the one hand, a religiously oriented answer might support the antiabortion argument. Suppose, for example, we said that a person consisted of a body combined with a soul, and suppose we also held that the soul combines with the body at the moment of conception. Then, clearly, a fetus is a person. On the other hand, a nonreligious answer might lead us to reject the claim that a fetus is a person. Suppose, for example, we held that an organism should not be counted as a person unless it is capable of thought, and suppose we held that a fetus could not think. Then we would have to say a fetus is not a person.

So, what is a person? If we want to say whether a fetus is a person, we need to answer this question. Our answer will be a nonreligious one since I think we can say what we mean by a *person* without bringing in religious ideas. Religiously minded people may disagree with this, and we will not argue that they are wrong. All we want to do here is give the best possible nonreligious account of what a person is.

It is best to begin our account of what a person is with an example which involves an old person instead of a fetus or an infant. So, consider an eighty-three-year-old woman who is becoming progressively more senile. First, her memory for dates and names begins to weaken and then to degenerate markedly. Then, her memory in general begins to decay. She confuses the past and the present, for example, sometimes insisting that her fifty-year-old daughter is only nineteen and about to come home from college for Christmas vacation. In general, the woman is losing her ability to think, plan, and act effectively. She also is losing her personality; that is, her characteristic feelings, emotions, perceptions, and interactions with others. Her personality is disintegrating as she becomes unable to think, plan, and act effectively. Despite all this the old woman is still a person.

What is it that makes the old woman still a person even as her personality disintegrates? To answer this question we need to note a simple fact; namely, each of us is the same person he was five years ago, ten years ago, twenty years ago, and so on. However much you have changed—even though your body changes and your beliefs, desires, attitudes, and emotions change—there is a sense in which you remain the same person. If you recall some event of your childhood, say, your eleventh birthday party, you are remembering the party which you—the person who now exists—had when that same person was eleven years old. There is, then, a sense in which you have remained the same person throughout your life. The concept of self-consciousness is the key to understanding this sense of the word *person.*

For me to be self-conscious is for me to be aware of *myself*, to be aware that *I* have certain experiences, thoughts, beliefs, desires, and the like, which we call *mental states*. Now, it is this "I" which remains the same person throughout changes in my body, my beliefs, desires, attitudes, and emotions. Philosophers have held various views about the nature of this "I." It has been suggested that the "I" is nothing over and above the stream of consciousness itself, the stream of thoughts, beliefs, desires, sensations. Alternatively, the "I" has been viewed as an entity which "contains" the stream of consciousness. The entity is sometimes thought of as the brain and sometimes as a completely nonphysical, purely mental entity. But whatever its nature, what we want to emphasize is that a person is an "I"—a self-conscious being. More precisely, *to be a person you must have mental states (like thoughts, beliefs, desires) and you must be capable of being aware of yourself as having such states.* Note that only the capacity for self-awareness is required here, not constant, actual awareness of yourself.

The old woman in our example is still a person by this definition. She still has mental states, and she is sometimes aware of herself as having such states. She may, for example, express awareness by saying such things as "I believe that my daughter will be home soon." A sentence like this expresses her consciousness of herself as having the belief in question. This example illustrates the fact that what the concept of a person does is distinguish between beings which are capable of self-awareness and those which are not. This distinction is important for morality, and, in fact, the distinction is crucial to the justification of abortion, as we will see in section 4.

One final philosophical qualification. While I think all of the preceding remarks are true of our concept of a person, I should point out that—strictly speaking—you can agree with what I say about abortion without agreeing with what I say about the concept of a person. As we will see, the crucial question for abortion is whether the fetus is a self-conscious being. Since I think a self-conscious being is a person, I translate this into the question of whether the fetus is a person. If you think I am wrong about what a person is, you should replace the word *person* in what follows by *self-conscious being*; all the arguments will still remain valid.

3. Is a fetus a person?

Now that we have settled on an account of what a person is, we can turn to the question of whether a fetus is a person since we now know what that question means. We know what we are asking is whether a fetus has mental states and whether it is capable of being aware of itself as having such states. There are two sources of relevant evidence.

The first source: behavioral evidence.   One way to determine whether a fetus has mental states and whether it is capable of being aware of itself as having such states is to look at behavior, for observing behavior can provide us with evidence that a being has mental states. It is worth illustrating this point by an example that does not involve fetuses or even human beings. Suppose we are watching a chimpanzee in a cage. There is a banana outside the cage beyond the chimp's reach. Inside the cage we have placed a stick which the chimp could use to reach the banana. We watch the chimp turn his head toward the banana, then turn his head toward the stick. After a few moments he suddenly rushes toward the stick, picks it up, and reaches for the banana. The natural explanation of this behavior is that the chimp *perceived* the banana, *perceived* the stick, and *realized* that he could reach the banana with the stick. Perceiving and realizing are mental states. We think the chimp has these states because his behavior (turning his head, rushing toward the stick) is evidence that he does; regarding the chimp as having these states allows us to explain his behavior.

Is there any behavioral evidence that a fetus has mental states? There is no single answer to this question. An answer must depend on how developed the fetus is. Consider the beginning of pregnancy. There is certainly no behavioral evidence at all that a fertilized ovum has any mental states whatsoever. It has no behavior which needs to be explained by regarding it as having beliefs, desires, emotions, perceptions, and so on. We can give a simpler explanation of what happens in the fertilized ovum without referring to mental states, and the simpler explanation here is to be preferred to the more complicated one. So, we should not regard the fertilized ovum as a person, and the antiabortion argument is certainly wrong when it insists that it is.

But suppose we turn our attention to the very end of pregnancy—in fact, to the newborn infant. Here there is rather clear behavioral evidence that the newborn infant has mental states, for the experience of pain is a mental state, and there is good evidence that a newborn infant experiences pain. Newborn infants struggle to avoid pinching, burning, scraping, poking, and so on, and they cry when they do so. We think what explains this behavior is the fact that pinching, burning, scraping, poking, and so on cause the newborn to experience pain. So, newborn infants have at least this mental state, and if newborn infants do then certainly fetuses very late in pregnancy do also. So, some fetuses have mental states, and this means they meet part of our requirement for being a person.

But do they meet all of that requirement? Recall what the definition of a person says: To be a person, you must have mental states, *and you must be capable of being aware of yourself as having those states.* Is a fetus or newborn infant capable of being aware of itself as having mental states? Is it capable of thinking, for example, "*I* am in pain"? What we want to know is whether the fetus or newborn can have thoughts which involve the concept of self—thoughts whose expression requires the use of the word *I*. We can begin by asking what behavior convinces us that adults have such thoughts.

It is linguistic behavior that convinces us, especially the use of the word *I*. For example, you think I have the concept of self because of the way I use sentences like the one you are now reading—sentences in which I use the word *I* to refer to myself. Of course, neither a fetus nor a newborn infant uses language at all, so we do not have any behavioral evidence that it has the concept of self. This does not mean it lacks that concept; all it means is that we have no behavioral evidence that it has it. To settle the question of whether a fetus or newborn has the concept of self we have to turn to the second of our two sources of evidence.

The second source: fetal development. Facts about the development of the nervous system provide us with our second source of evidence. What we want to look at is the development in the fetus of the cerebral cortex—the convoluted grey matter of the brain—because a fetus is a developing human being, and in human beings thought and consciousness coincide with activity in the cerebral cortex.[5] This last statement can be easily misunderstood. It does not mean that thought is only brain activity, nor does it mean that brain activity causes thought; rather, it says the two go together—in human beings.

The fact to emphasize is that without activity in the cortex a human being does not think and is not conscious. So, since activity in the cortex is required for thought and consciousness in general, it is required for the particular sort of thought we are interested in—thoughts whose expression in language requires the use of *I*. Is a fetus' cortex developed enough for thought and consciousness to occur? Here are the relevant facts.

The cerebral cortex consists of ten billion nerve cells called neurons.[6] After six months almost all these neurons are present in the brain of a fetus. But this does not mean that a fetal cortex is sufficiently developed for thought to occur. In an adult, developed cortex the ten billion neurons are interconnected in a very intricate pattern; on the average, a single neuron is connected to ten thousand others. In the fetal brain these connections are virtually nonexistent. In fact, they are only gradually established in the first two years after birth.[7] This is a very important fact, for the interconnections of the neurons are essential to the occurrence of thought and consciousness.[8]

Thought and consciousness, therefore, do not occur in a fetus or even in a newborn infant. So, since it cannot think, a fetus or newborn cannot have thoughts whose expression would require the use of the word *I*. And this means that neither a fetus nor a newborn counts as a person. Of course, it is a potential person; that is, it is an organism of the sort which normally develops into a person, but it is not yet a person. The antiabortion argument is wrong, then, when it assumes that a fetus is a person, and so we have shown that the argument rests on a false premise. But we have not yet shown that abortion is justified. To do we have to develop a proabortion argument. We needed to criticize the antiabortion argument first, however, since the proabortion argument will rest on the assumption that a fetus is not a person, but only a potential person.

4. A proabortion argument

We can begin our proabortion argument by questioning the assumption that no circumstances justify overriding the fetus' right to consent. There is good reason to question it, for in making that assumption the antiabortion argument is also implicitly assuming that the right to consent of the pregnant woman who wants an abortion is always justifiably overridden. In fact, the implicit assumption here involves more than the right to consent. What is fundamentally involved is the woman's right to self-determination (the right from which the right to consent is derived).

To see this, consider the case of Karen. Rape is a violent and brutal interference with Karen's—and any woman's—life, mind, and body. It violates her right to self-determination in a vicious and barbaric way, and a pregnancy resulting from the rape is a continuation of this violation. If Karen has the child, her plans and projects will be forcibly and drastically altered—at least for the nine months of pregnancy and for much longer if she keeps the child. Why should anyone have to suffer such a violation of the right to self-determination?

The antiabortion argument would have us believe that the fetus should be allowed to develop even at the cost of sacrificing the actual ongoing plans of the pregnant woman. This is the effect of assuming that nothing overrides the right to consent of the fetus.

The proabortion argument, of course, sees the situation quite differently. The basic claim of the proabortion argument is that *the woman's right to self-determination justifies abortion in certain cases—* pregnancy as a result of rape being such a case. The proabortion point of view emphasizes the fact that abortion protects the woman's plans and projects, and the question the proabortion argument must answer is why doing this is worth stopping the development of the fetus. And it is not easy to answer this question since it is possible to make a good case in favor of letting the fetus develop. To see this, consider that each of us has a reason to maximize self-realization. We argued for this in the Introduction,[9] and we have appealed to this fact repeatedly through the last two chapters. Now, wouldn't letting the fetus live and develop increase the overall amount of self-realization? The fetus will develop into a person capable of self-realization, and so it will add the total self-realization it experiences to the overall amount of self-realization. Of course, if the woman—like Karen—does not want the child, her self-realization will be adversely affected. She will experience less self-realization than she would if she had an abortion—unless, of course, she comes to enjoy raising the child. But, even if that does not happen, won't it be true—in most cases, at least—that the woman's loss of self-realization is more than made up by the amount of self-realization experienced by the fetus? After all, we are weighing the total self-realization of the entire life of the person the fetus would develop into against the woman's loss of self-realization over having an unwanted child. The woman's loss may be great, but certainly it is not as great as the total amount of self-realization that we can reasonably expect a person to experience in an entire lifetime. So, there is a good reason to let the fetus live and develop, the reason being that doing so helps maximize self-realization.

We should recognize the fact that this is a good reason against abortion. It helps explain why abortion worries us, and why we feel it needs justification. It helps us see why a person might hold the anti-abortion position and think that nothing should be allowed to override the fetus' right to consent. Still, we want to emphasize the proabortion argument claims that the woman's right to self-determination outweighs the reason we have to let the fetus develop—at least in certain cases.

The clearest way to present the proabortion argument is to look again at the case of Karen. We want to ask two questions—one about Karen and one about the fetus. Then we want to compare the answers, for the comparison will show us that the abortion is justified—even given the reason (maximizing self-realization) which we have for letting the fetus develop.

The first question is: Would denying her the abortion violate any of Karen's rights? We have already answered this question, for we have seen that denying Karen the abortion violates both her right to consent and her right to self-determination. Abortion is a medical procedure to which Karen certainly has the right to consent. If she requests an abortion and is denied it, her right to consent has been violated. Denying her the abortion also violates her right to self-determination since it interferes—in a drastic way—with her plans and projects.

The second question is: Would aborting the fetus violate any of its rights? I think the answer must be *no*. We will explain this answer in three steps. First, we will argue that the right to consent is not violated by abortion. Second, we will argue the same for the right to self-determination, and third, we will consider whether abortion violates any other rights.

The right to consent. To see that abortion does not violate the fetus' right to consent, recall the full statement of the right to consent, which we gave in Chapter 1.[10] *The right to consent is the right to give or withhold consent to any action which has a significant chance of interfering with our pursuit of self-realization.* Now, if abortion violates the fetus' right to consent, it must therefore interfere with the fetus' pursuit of self-realization. Does it? No, it cannot possibly do so since the fetus is not the kind of being capable of self-realization. To be capable of self-realization, we must have an ideal self-image since to achieve self-realization is to act in ways that are motivated by, and which conform to, our ideal self-image. But to have a self-image we must have a conception of how we would most like to be. Now, such a conception is a form of self-awareness, and self-awareness is something the fetus is not capable of. We made this point in the last section when we argued that a fetus is not a person but only a potential person.

Our conclusion, then, is that the fetus is not capable of self-realization, and that because of this abortion cannot count as a violation of its right to consent. In fact, since abortion cannot ever be a violation of the fetus' right to consent, it would be clearer to say that the fetus does not have the right to consent to abortion.

But perhaps it is irrelevant that abortion does not violate the fetus' right to consent. Perhaps we should consider the right to consent of the person the fetus could become. Doesn't abortion possibly violate that person's right to consent? The issues raised by this question are rather theoretical, so we will treat them in the section on theoretical foundations. There we will argue that it is impossible to violate the rights of a person who never will exist (how can you possibly interfere with what does not exist?). So, since abortion ensures that the person the fetus could be will never exist, abortion cannot violate that person's rights.

The right to self-determination. Abortion does not violate the fetus' right to self-determination for the same reason it does not violate its right to consent. Recall that the right to self-determination is the right to pursue those plans and projects we believe will lead to our self-realization. Since a fetus is not the sort of being capable of self-realization, abortion cannot interfere with its pursuit of those plans and projects it believes will lead to its self-realization. A fetus is not even capable of having beliefs about self-realization. So, abortion does not violate a fetus' right to self-determination. And, again, we do not have to worry about violating the right to self-determination of the person the fetus could have become because we cannot violate the rights of a person who will never exist.

Other rights.   Perhaps abortion violates some right of the fetus other than the right to consent and the right to self-determination, such as the right to life. In a way abortion does violate the right to life. Recall that to say the fetus has a right to life is to say that each person has a reason (of a certain special sort) not to interfere with its living, and we have already said we do have a reason—namely, maximizing self-realization—to let the fetus live and develop. So, we already recognize something like a right to life, but we will argue that this reason for letting the fetus develop can be outweighed by other reasons which favor abortion. In general, what one needs to consider in discussing abortion is determined by one's theoretical framework. Given our theoretical framework, the only rights we need to consider are the right to self-determination and the right to consent, for we have taken the right to self-determination as basic and fundamental. We will assume, then, that there are no other rights of the fetus which might possibly be violated by abortion. Therefore, the answer to our second question is *no*, abortion does not violate any right of the fetus. Nor does it violate any right of the person the fetus could become.

If we put the answers to the above two questions together, we get a justification of abortion in Karen's case. Look at it this way. What is the cost of not aborting? If we deny Karen the abortion we violate her rights, interfere with her plans, and make her suffer. The quality of her self-realization will decrease in the sense that she will get less of what she most wants. Now, what is the cost of aborting? The cost is that we lose all the self-realization represented by the fetus. But, on the plus side, we respect Karen's rights, her plans and projects, and the quality of her self-realization. And, we gain this without violating any right of the fetus or of the person the fetus could become. In addition, there are always ways to compensate for the loss of self-realization represented by the aborted fetus. For example, by aborting the fetus we preserve Karen's freedom to have other children when she chooses and with whom she chooses. We also preserve her freedom to expend her energy on increasing her own self-realization or the self-realization of others. The case for abortion is clearly the stronger one here. We ought to protect the quality of Karen's self-realization at the cost of aborting the fetus.

We have justified abortion in one case—the case of pregnancy as a result of rape. In the next section we will generalize the conclusions we have reached so that they apply to other cases.

5. The Quality Principle

In Karen's case we decided that the quality of her self-realization should not be sacrificed by letting the fetus develop. What convinced us this was true was basically the degree to which the quality of her life would be affected. We can generalize from our reasoning about Karen to the following principle, which we will call the Quality Principle:

The quality of self-realization of any existing person should not be sacrificed—*to any significant degree*—simply in order to allow a potential person to develop.

What counts as a "significant degree?" There is no general answer to this question, but we can illustrate what is involved by means of examples. We will consider five cases.

First case. Suppose a woman will die as a result of her pregnancy unless she has an abortion. If she does not have the abortion, the quality of self-realization is certainly destroyed since a futile pregnancy resulting in death puts an end to all her attempts to realize her self-image. This is a clear case in which the Quality Principle justifies abortion. Here the degree is certainly significant.

Second case. Consider a case at the opposite end of the spectrum. Suppose a husband wants his wife to have an abortion simply because he does not like the way she looks when she is pregnant. Even granting that the difference in looks will affect the quality of the man's self-realization, we should not use the Quality Principle to justify abortion here (even if his wife is willing). The reason for the abortion is too trivial, too weak; it does not defeat the reason—maximizing self-realization—we have for letting the fetus develop. Of course, it is possible to imagine a complicated case in which the way the wife looked so affected the couple's self-realization that an abortion was justified. But here the degree is insignificant.

Third case. We began the chapter with this case. Suppose a woman and her husband both decide they want a child, and so the woman becomes pregnant. But now confronted with the daily fact of pregnancy, they change their minds and decide they are not yet ready to raise a child. Is abortion justified? The problem here is to determine the degree to which the quality of their self-realization would be affected by having the child. It is difficult to figure out just what this degree is since we have only their word that they are not ready to raise a child. Perhaps they are wrong about this; perhaps their decision is simply the result of losing confidence in their ability to be good parents. On the other hand, suppose they are right; suppose they really are not ready to raise a child and that doing so would result in a severe emotional strain on their marriage. Would this be a sufficient decrease in the quality of their self-realization to justify abortion? I think so, but there are no simple rules which tell us how to evaluate such cases. Each of us has to rely on his or her own personal judgment. The fourth case—a birth defect case—also illustrates the difficulty of determining when the degree is significant.

Fourth case.   Many birth defects can be detected early enough in pregnancy by the procedure of amniocentesis to make abortion medically feasible. Down's syndrome—or mongolism—is one such defect. Suppose the fetus you are carrying has been found to be mongoloid. Would you abort it? When you got pregnant you did so with the idea of having a normal, healthy, happy child. You do not want a mongoloid child. Having a mongoloid child would be contrary to your expectations and desires. Still, you know that, unless the degree of retardation is severe, mongoloid children can live happy lives. Is the interference with the quality of your life sufficient to justify the abortion? I think so, but you must answer this question for yourself.

Fifth case.   Lesch-Nyhan syndrome is another birth defect which can be detected early enough in pregnancy to make abortion feasible. This defect results in severe mental retardation, uncontrollable aggression, and self-mutilation. The Quality Principle certainly justifies abortions of this sort since children with Lesch-Nyhan syndrome are generally a great emotional and financial strain on their families. The point we should emphasize here is that the Quality Principle would also justify infanticide—killing the infant after it is born. The reason for this is that the argument we have for abortion is also an argument for infanticide, which is that the newborn infant is—like a fetus—only a potential person. So, we could just repeat the abortion argument to argue for infanticide. We would just replace the word *fetus* with *newborn* and *abort* with *kill.*

This is perhaps surprising. Most people find infanticide more objectionable than abortion, but according to our position each can be equally well justified. So why do we react differently? It is easy to see why, if you imagine killing an infant. The infant is alive and breathing, living "on its own." Killing it is much more immediate than aborting a fetus, and so we are more reluctant to do it. It runs counter to our respect for life. Indeed, I am not sure that I, for one, could bring myself to do it—even if I was convinced it was necessary. Still, infanticide can be justified in certain cases. Suppose, for example, that Lesch-Nyhan syndrome had not been detected during pregnancy but only after birth. Then, I think, the Quality Principle would justify infanticide. (Of course, killing the infant would be illegal; this is one clear point where our moral reasoning does not agree with the law.)

This fifth case raises another point worth discussing. In the case of a defect as severe as Lesch-Nyhan, many think it is true that the life of the person the fetus would become *is not a life worth living because it is too full of pain and suffering,* and so they think the fetus should be aborted (or the newborn infant killed). Here, we are appealing to the quality of life of a *future* person to justify abortion. This is quite different than what we do when we apply the Quality Principle. When we apply that principle, we look at the quality of life of people *who already exist.* What we are suggesting now is that it is sometimes relevant to evaluate the quality of life of a person who does not yet exist and who may never exist. The idea is that, if the future life of a potential person is not worth living, then that potential person should not be allowed to develop. This idea should be discussed at some length, and we will do so in the next section where we will switch our focus from abortion to infanticide. The point of switching our focus to infanticide is that the question of whether it is permissible to kill a newborn infant often arises because someone is convinced that the future life of the infant will not be worth living. Of course, if we decide that infanticide is permissible because the infant's future life will not be worth living, then the same sort of argument could also be used to justify abortion.

6. Infanticide and health

Suppose you give birth to an infant who has Lesch-Nyhan syndrome. To amplify the definition we gave in the last section, Lesch-Nyhan is a neurological disease characterized by cerebral palsy, involuntary muscle movement, mental retardation, aggression, and compulsive biting which results in self-mutilation of the lips and fingers. The infant also has another defect besides Lesch-Nyhan. It has no opening between the stomach and the small intestine (duodenum). This means it cannot be fed normally, and this defect must be corrected if it is to live. You refuse to consent to the operation which would repair this defect and request instead that the infant be allowed to die. Your doctor agrees with this request and arranges for the infant to die of starvation in the nursery.

You and your doctor have committed infanticide. Can your action be justified? If the child would be a severe financial and emotional burden on the family, we could use the Quality Principle to justify infanticide. But what we are interested in here is a different sort of justification—one which focuses on the quality of life the infant will have. Now, in fact, many people think that infanticide is permissible in cases of birth defects as severe as Lesch-Nyhan, and they hold this because they think the infant's future life is not worth living. The basic issue is proxy consent. What we are doing is deciding *on behalf of a person who could exist* that his life is not worth living. Can we justify consenting to death on behalf of a person because we judge his future life to be not worth living? Let us answer this question first for the particular example described above. As the antiabortion argument pointed out, (P2) is the principle which applies in cases of proxy consent involving potential persons. Now, in the particular case at hand, (P2)—when combined with facts about the quality of the infant's future life—makes infanticide *morally obligatory*. Applied to this case (P2) says that

> with respect to the infant, we should perform those therapeutic actions, and only those therapeutic actions, which maintain its physical and mental health.

"Health" here is to be understood to mean overall health (Chapter 2, section 6). What we are claiming is that the operation to repair the infant's intestinal defect will not maintain the infant's overall health. The reason is that the future life of the particular infant we are considering contains no possibility of self-realization; so therefore the infant has no overall health.[11] Hence, the operation cannot possibly contribute to its overall health. In such a situation (P2) rules out the operation, for (P2) says we should perform those—and only those— actions which maintain the infant's (overall) health.

It is important to note here that (P2) rules out infanticide in cases which are not as severe as the one described. If anything can be done to maintain the infant's overall health, (P2) requires that we do it. *So, a consideration of the quality of the infant's future life justifies infanticide (and likewise abortion) only in the most extreme cases.* In all other cases we must appeal instead to the Quality Principle.

Another important point to note here is that when (P2) does make infanticide obligatory, what it requires us to do is let the infant die. As we noted in Chapter 2, (P2) rules out killing. However, if we are convinced in a particular case that (P2) requires us to let an infant die, the moral (although not the legal) thing to do is to kill it. That will spare the infant the pain and suffering of a lingering death.

7. Conclusion

We have justified abortion and infanticide in certain cases. The crucial claim in our argument was that a fetus or newborn was not a person. If you disagree with this claim, you should work out your own alternative and your own position on abortion and infanticide. The claim that a fetus or newborn is not yet a person certainly does not mean we can do as we please with it. For example, suppose that, for no other reason than maliciousness, we maim a fetus we know will not be aborted. Even if we maim it painlessly, it is still wrong to do so. One reason it is wrong is that by maiming it we interfere with the right to self-determination of the person it will become. That person will be less able to pursue his or her self-realization. So, those fetuses and newborns who will be allowed to develop are protected by the rights of the person they will become.

THEORETICAL FOUNDATIONS

We have one problem left over: Why is it impossible to violate the rights of a person who never will exist? This question arose in section 4 when we claimed that abortion did not violate the rights of the person the fetus could become. Why is this claim true? To see why it is true, we first need to ask what it is to violate someone's rights. To violate someone's rights is to interfere with them in some way, and to interfere is to act in a way that prevents or hinders—or might reasonably be expected to prevent or hinder—a person from doing what he wants or getting what he needs. In other words, interference is interference with a person's desires or needs.

Now we obviously cannot interfere with the desires of a person who will never exist, for if the person will never exist his desires do not exist for us to interfere with. Even keeping the person from coming into existence (by abortion, say) cannot count as interference with his desires because keeping the person from coming into existence ensures that his desires will not exist. It ensures that there will be no desires of that person with which we can interfere.

Perhaps we can interfere with the needs of a person who will never exist. But how? How can a person who will never exist need anything? Since he will never exist, he has no goals, desires, or plans for which he would need things. Also, it makes no sense to talk of a person who will never exist as needing to exist. Since the person will never exist, there is no one with this need.

Therefore, since we cannot interfere with the desires or needs of a person who will never exist, we cannot violate the rights of a person who will never exist.

A FURTHER QUESTION

A woman who has one hemophiliac child is pregnant again. She wants another child, but she definitely does not want another hemophiliac child. She cannot afford it, she says; she can accept neither the financial burden nor the emotional strain. Unfortunately, hemophilia is an inheritable disease, a fact of which she was aware before she became pregnant. Women do not suffer from it, but they may carry the genetic trait for it, and a carrier—like the woman in our example—has a 50-50 chance of transmitting the disease to her male offspring. Also, there is a 50-50 chance that her female offspring will be carriers. What should this woman do? There is no test for hemophilia prior to birth, so the woman has just four options: (1) have the child; (2) have the child and put it up for adoption; (3) determine the sex of the child (by amniocentesis) and abort all males; or (4) wait until the child is born and have it killed if it has hemophilia.

The woman has made up her mind against (1). (2) might be a difficult alternative to take. Who is going to adopt a hemophiliac child? (3) means having a 50-50 chance of aborting a healthy male fetus. (4) involves all the problems and emotions surrounding the issue of infanticide. It also means going through an entire pregnancy without knowing whether you will have a child to love or a defective infant to kill. Which alternative should the woman take?

NOTES

1. See Albert R. Johnson and Michael J. Garland, "A Moral Policy: Life/Death Decisions in the Intensive Care Nursery," *Medical Dimensions,* Vol. 6, No. 4 (April 1977), pp. 27-35.
2. See Chapter 1, section 5 for a discussion of proxy consent.
3. See Chapter 1, pp. 34-35.
4. The next section argues at length for this claim.
5. This statement is intended to be compatible with any reasonable position on the interaction of the mental and the physical. The claim that thought and activity in the cerebral cortex coincide is one for which we have a great deal of evidence. Even so, it is worth pointing out that all the arguments of this and the next two sections could rest on the weaker claim that cerebral cortex activity coincides with self-awareness.
6. See Edmund S. Crelin, Ph.D., D.Se., *Development of the Nervous System, Clinical Symposia,* Vol. 26, No. 2 (1974).
7. Crelin, *Development of the Nervous System,* p. 18.

8. The reason the interconnections are essential is that the nervous system uses a spatio-temporal code to manipulate information. The spatial interconnections are essential to the use of this code. (See Richard Mark, *Memory and Nerve Cell Connection,* New York: Oxford University Press, 1974, pp. 16–20.) Unless information is manipulated in this way, thought and consciousness do not occur in human beings.
9. Introduction, p. 15.
10. Chapter 1, p. 18.
11. Lesch-Nyhan syndrome can occur with varying degrees of severity. Let us suppose we are dealing with a severe case so that it is clear that the infant's future life holds no possibility of self-realization. I am indebted to Dr. Gary Glass, M.D. for this point.

BIBLIOGRAPHY

General

Callahan, Daniel. *Abortion. Law, Choice and Morality.* New York: Macmillan, 1970.
Thompson, Judith Jarvis. "A Defense of Abortion." *Philosophy and Public Affairs,* Vol. 1, No. 1, Fall 1971. Pp. 47–66. (Also reprinted in David Berlinski. *Philossophy: The Cutting Edge.* Sherman Oaks, Calif.: Alfred, 1976. Pp. 465–480.)
Tooley, Michael. "A Defense of Abortion and Infanticide." *Philosophy and Public Affairs,* Vol. 2, No. 1, Fall 1971. Pp. 37–65.

Religious perspectives

Feldman, David, M. *Birth Control in Jewish Law.* New York: New York University Press, 1968.
Noonan, John T., Jr. ed. *The Morality of Abortion.* Cambridge, Mass.: Harvard University Press, 1970.

FOUR

Mental Disorders:
Moral and Legal Issues

Consent, definition, and deviance. These are the headings under which we can classify the three main moral problems raised by psychiatry and psychotherapy. Problems about consent arise because it is often impossible for a therapist's patient to give or withhold free and informed consent to his treatment; for example, when the patient is too mentally disordered for his consent to count as either free or informed. In such situations, the therapist decides what is best for his patient; in effect, the therapist gives consent to treatment on behalf of his patient. We need to determine whether this is justified; and if we decide that it is, we need to formulate a principle of proxy consent[1] which safeguards a psychiatric patient's right to consent.[2]

The problem of definition is the problem of defining mental disorders. When we define a mental disorder we are saying that the people who fit the definition are unhealthy because of the way in which they think, feel, and act; and to say this is to say in part that they would be better off if they thought, felt, and acted differently than they do.[3] So, in giving such definitions we may be imposing our views about how to live on people who may not share them. Can we justify this? This question is especially important because of the connection between the problem of definition and the problem of consent. When we find that a person is mentally disordered, we tend to regard this as evidence that he may be incapable of giving or withholding free and informed consent. Consequently, definitions of mental disorders have implications for how we will treat the right to consent of people who fit the definition.

Finally, there is the problem of deviance. Deviant individuals are people who are socially maladjusted or psychologically abnormal. Some deviants are harmless, such as the senile old lady who wanders the streets followed by her cat. But child molesters and mass murderers are obviously a totally different matter. The question is: Should we use therapy, drugs, and psychosurgery to control the behavior of deviant people? In particular, to control the behavior of deviants who are likely to harm others? If so, when and how? The issues raised by deviance clearly combine the problems of consent and definition. The problem of consent arises because we will often need to override the right to consent of a deviant person if we want to control his behavior, and the problem of definition arises because what we count as deviant is determined, at least in part, by what we count as a mental disorder.

We will take up the problems of consent, definition, and deviance in that order. First, however, it is worthwhile to consider examples of all three problems, for this will give us a good overview of the issues.

1. Issues and examples

We will begin with two examples which illustrate the problems associated with the right to consent.

Example 1. Mr. Miller is a successful, middle-aged lawyer who has just been admitted to the emergency room of a hospital after attempting suicide by taking a massive dose of barbiturates. A friend who came by his house found him unconscious and rushed him to the hospital where the resident on call responded immediately to the medical emergency. Since time mattered, he did not bother to get consent from anyone.[4]

A staff psychiatrist who talks to Miller two days later discovers that he tried to kill himself because he was depressed about the recent death of his wife in an auto accident. Since they had no children and relied heavily on each other for companionship, her sudden and unexpected death was a severe emotional shock which threw Miller into a profound depression, a depression from which he has not yet recovered. The psychiatrist thinks Miller definitely should have short-term therapy to pull him through this period of depression. However, he does not say so directly to Miller; instead, he approaches the issue of therapy carefully, and he deliberately but subtly manipulates Miller into arranging to see one of the three psychiatrists whose names and telephone numbers he gives him.[5] The psychiatrist is virtually certain—from what he had already learned from Miller's friends, his doctor, and the nurses— that Miller would refuse therapy if it were openly suggested, for Miller's depression is still making everything look hopeless.

In this example, Miller's right to consent is overridden twice. The first violation occurs when he arrives at the hospital. Since Miller was unconscious then, he was unable to give or withhold free and informed consent to the actions taken to save his life. Now, given that Miller really had his mind set on suicide, he might very well have refused to consent to having his life saved if he had been conscious and able to give or withhold consent. Let us suppose this was so—that, had he been conscious, Miller would have refused treatment. In fact, we can further suppose that the friend who brought Miller to the hospital knew Miller had firmly made up his mind to kill himself (and had come to Miller's house to try to talk him out of it).

Given these circumstances, saving Miller's life clearly overrides his right to consent. Not violating his right to consent would mean following (P1), the principle of proxy consent which applies when there is someone present—like the friend in this case—who knows what the patient would decide if he were capable of giving free and informed consent. Applied to this case, (P1) says:

We ought to consent on Miller's behalf to saving his life if and only if we have good reason to think that Miller would consent to this if he were capable of giving free and informed consent.

Now, Miller's friend certainly does not have "good reason to think that Miller would consent" to having his life saved. On the contrary, he knows Miller would refuse. So, by saving Miller's life his friend and doctor violate his right to consent. The reason the friend acts as he does is that he assumes Miller really wants to live. He thinks this desire is still there in Miller but that Miller does not realize it, for his depression has made everything look so hopeless that he is convinced life is no longer worth living. Of course, the friend could be wrong about this, but—for the purposes of our example—let us suppose he is right, that Miller really wants to live.

We said Miller's right to consent was overridden twice, and it is the psychiatrist who violates it the second time. He does it by influencing Miller's decision to have short-term therapy. By manipulating Miller into this decision, he overrides his right to give or withhold *free* and informed consent, for a decision so strongly influenced should not be counted as free.

Can we justify these violations of Miller's right to consent? Most of us probably think so. At least, most of us probably think the first violation—saving Miller's life—is justified. Miller's decision to commit suicide was made in a state of severe depression, and we tend to think this fact gives us a strong reason to override the right to consent in order to save his life. But why? And if Miller's depression justifies overriding his right to consent to save his life, does it also justify the psychiatrist's violation of his right to consent? We will consider such issues in sections 2 and 3. Section 2 focuses on the general issue of overriding a mentally disturbed person's right to consent. Section 3 contains a detailed examination of Miller's case.

Example 2. We have seen that a psychiatrist's manipulation can violate the right to consent. This sort of manipulation is a constant feature of psychiatry and psychotherapy. Consider the following example taken from an actual case.[6]

A husband and wife have come to see a therapist because their child is terrified of dogs. The boy's fear is so great that he is unwilling to go outside the house, and when he is outside he will even run into traffic to avoid a dog. The boy's dog phobia is the problem the parents want treated. The therapist quickly realizes that the problem they want treated is only a reflection of the basic underlying problem which is the parents' relationship. The parents relate to each other only through the boy; they are otherwise cut off from each other, living almost totally separate lives. This situation has arisen because of a long-standing, un-resolved marital problem, and their son has become the focal point for his parents' marital difficulties and tensions. His dog phobia is just a reflection of the tensions which the parents work out through him, and the therapist sees that if he can get the parents to resolve their problem, the dog phobia will disappear.

So, the therapist begins to meet regularly with both the parents and the boy. He sees that the mother is intensely involved with the boy. She hovers over him, finishes his sentences for him, and generally thrusts on him the opinions she thinks he ought to have. The father, on the other hand, is detached and uninvolved. Confronted with this situation, the therapist decides to pry the mother apart from her son while bring-ing the father in closer contact with him. And he also decides to involve the parents more directly with each other—an understandable decision given his conception of the basic problem. He accomplishes these goals indirectly by a variety of techniques which he uses to manipulate the interactions of the family as they talk with him and with each other. (By the way, in the actual case these techniques proved equal to the task. The dog phobia disappeared, and the parents resolved their marital problem.)

The one thing the therapist does not do is tell the parents what the problem really is and what he is doing about it.[7] The parents are treated in a way to which they have not consented for a problem which is different than the one for which they have explicitly requested treatment. This is a violation of their right to give or withhold free and informed consent. It is useful to compare the psychiatrist's actions in this case with what the psychiatrist did in Miller's case. With Miller, the psychiatrist's manipulations violated his freedom; they violated his right to give *free* and informed consent. In this case, the emphasis is on infor-mation instead of freedom. The therapist's hidden manipulations over-ride the parents' right to give free and *informed* consent. In general, psychiatric manipulation can violate the right to consent in either or both of these ways.

Can we justify overriding the right to consent in these ways? This question is one of the most important and far reaching we can raise, for concealed manipulation is a feature of virtually all psychiatry and psychotherapy, and it is easy to see why. People generally tend to resist overt manipulation, so it makes sense for a therapist to conceal his manipulations since they will be more effective if they are not out in the open. Consider, for example, what might have happened if Miller's psychiatrist had straightforwardly tried to talk Miller into therapy. Imagine the psychiatrist saying something like, "In my experience, people generally recover from even such a severe emotional loss as yours, and short-term therapy is often useful in this process." This might have convinced Miller, but it is likely he would have just insisted that his life was no longer worth living. Such a straightforward approach rarely alters a severely depressed person's point of view. Similarly, imagine what would have happened in the dog phobia case if the therapist had said to the parents, "The basic problem is not your son's dog phobia. The problem is with you two. You relate to each other only through your son." The parents might have refused therapy since they might not have agreed that the basic problem was a marital one. Or even if they had agreed and consented to therapy, the fact that they knew what the therapist was aiming at might well have made the therapy much less effective. So, it is clearly crucial to determining our attitude toward psychotherapy to know whether we can justify the violation of the right to consent by concealed psychiatric manipulation.

Example 3.   Let us turn from problems about consent to the problem of definition. Consider the following definition of the schizoid personality given in the *Diagnostic and Statistical Manual of Mental Disorders:*

> This behavior pattern manifests shyness, oversensitivity, seclusiveness, avoidance of close or competitive relationships, and often eccentricity. Autistic thinking without loss of capacity to recognize reality is common, as are daydreaming and the inability to express hostility and ordinary aggressive feelings. These patients react to disturbing experiences and conflicts with apparent detachment.[8]

This is a description of a type of personality. By including this description in a manual of mental disorders, we are claiming that any person who fits this description is *unhealthy* because of the way in which he acts, thinks, and feels, and therefore that the person would be better off if he thought, felt, and acted differently than he does. To justify the definition of a mental disorder, we have to justify these claims. Section 4 takes up this issue.

We will also consider in that section the link between the problem of definition and the problems of consent—why we tend to regard the fact that a person is mentally disordered as evidence that he may not be capable of giving free and informed consent. The preceding definition of the schizoid personality illustrates the issue. A schizoid personality exhibits autistic thinking; in other words, he is overly focused on his own subjective mental states, engages (perhaps) in wish-fulfillment fantasies, and generally ignores external reality. Is such a person capable of giving or withholding free and informed consent to psychiatric treatment? Perhaps—it will depend on the circumstances; but his autistic thinking is evidence that he *may* not be able to. Why is this so?

Example 4. Finally, there is the issue of deviance. Mass killers and child molesters are dramatic examples of deviant individuals; however, it will be useful here to focus on a less sensational but more common form of deviance. Kelly is a fifty-year-old vagrant. In warm weather he sleeps in an abandoned house. In cold weather he usually sleeps over a large steam vent outside a hospital—a habit which earned him the nickname "vent-man" with the hospital staff. Kelly is psychotic but basically harmless. He hears voices and has conversations with imaginary people whom he hallucinates. Occasionally, he shouts at passersby and sometimes he will stand motionless in the middle of a busy street. If he shouts enough or blocks enough traffic, the police will pick him up and bring him to the emergency room of the nearest hospital. If he is extremely agitated he will probably be admitted to the hospital for a few days, given some drugs to calm him down, and then (if he wants) released.

What is happening here is that the police and the hospital cooperate in controlling Kelly's deviant behavior so that it is not too disruptive. This is the point of the hospitalization and the drug therapy. The aim is not to cure but to control. There cannot be any other realistic aim since the prognosis for a well-established psychosis like Kelly's is extremely poor. The issue here is: Should we use the techniques of psychiatry and psychotherapy—drugs, therapy, and psychosurgery—to control the behavior of deviant people? If so, when and how? Section 5 takes up these questions.

2. Overriding the right to consent: irrationality

When are we justified in overriding the right to consent because a person is mentally disordered? Consider the case of Miller again. His decision to commit suicide was made in a state of severe depression, and most of us probably think this justifies overriding his right to consent in order to save his life. But why? The answer, I think, must be as follows. First, we have a strong reason to override a person's right to consent when he is sufficiently irrational. And second, Miller's severe state of depression is evidence of a sufficient degree of irrationality. Both parts of this answer raise further questions. What do we mean by irrationality? And what counts as a sufficient degree of irrationality? Before we can take up these questions, however, we must focus on the fundamental issue of why a sufficient degree of irrationality gives us a reason to override a person's right to consent. It is helpful to begin with an example.

Mason's case.   Mason, a twenty-one-year-old university student, was brought into the emergency room after the police found him running naked down one of the city's main streets threatening to kill anyone who got in his way. The psychiatrist discovers that Mason feels his thoughts, impulses, and actions are controlled by beings from outer space—the Zircons. He has no choice but to submit passively to their commands, commands which, he insists, the Zircons communicate to him by mental telepathy. He hears their voices in his head, and he also broadcasts thoughts to them. Sometimes they also send him messages over TV. It turns out that the Zircons commanded him to run naked down the street—just as they are now commanding him to leave the hospital. Mason insists he does not know how he got to the hospital or why he is there, but he is determined to leave, and he shouts out that if anyone tries to stop him he will kill everyone in the hospital with the special mental death-ray the Zircons have given him.

Mason does not succeed in leaving, however. Since he assaulted the two police officers who brought him in, the psychiatrist decides that Mason is genuinely violent and a danger to others—if not also to himself. So, on these grounds Mason is committed to the hospital against his will for seventy-two hours. Being a danger to oneself or others is the typical reason for the involuntary commitment of a mentally disordered person. It is the reason generally recognized by the courts.[9] However, from a moral point of view, what is crucial to justifying Mason's involuntary commitment is his irrationality.

Justification.   To see the justification, recall that, as we saw in Chapter 1,[10] the basic reason for respecting a person's right to consent is to help maximize free, rational choice, and the reason we want to maximize free, rational choice is that doing so is what best promotes self-realization. *But*—and this is the point to emphasize here—this reason does not apply in Mason's case because Mason is irrational. Why should Mason be regarded as irrational,[11] and why does this take away the usual reason we have for respecting the right to consent?

Mason is irrational because he makes no attempt to base his decisions and actions on adequate information about himself and his environment. Instead, his decisions and actions are the result of the voices he hears, voices which express opinions and commands generated by Mason's own disordered mental state. Because of Mason's irrationality he cannot effectively pursue his own self-realization. To pursue self-realization effectively, we have to be able to gain and use accurate information about our environment; otherwise our attempts at self-realization will be based on unrealistic assumptions and will (most likely) end in failure. But gaining and using accurate information about his environment is just what Mason is currently incapable of doing. So, respecting Mason's right to consent will not help promote self-realization by maximizing free, rational choice—since Mason is not capable of rational choice. This means the reason we normally have for respecting the right to consent does not apply.

In fact, it is overriding Mason's right to consent which promotes self-realization in this case. We increase Mason's chances for self-realization by committing him against his will; not only do we keep Mason from harming himself, we also create the possibility of using drugs and therapy to make him more capable of dealing effectively with himself and his environment. In addition, we also keep Mason from interfering violently with the plans and projects of others as they pursue their self-realization.

Generalizing from Mason's case, we can say that a sufficient degree of irrationality—a degree as extreme as Mason's, for example—provides us with a strong reason to override the right to consent. This happens because the basic reason we have to respect the right to consent does not apply, and because overriding the right to consent is what is most likely to promote self-realization. Now, even a degree of irrationality as extreme as Mason's does not automatically justify overriding the right to consent; it just provides a strong reason for doing so, but there may, in any given case, be better reasons for not doing so. Suppose, for example, the psychiatrist was able to contact some of Mason's friends who then came to the hospital. They inform the psychiatrist that Mason had been seeing a psychiatrist in his hometown in the summer, and that they are sure his parents would like to have him come home and be treated by that psychiatrist. A phone call to the parents verifies this information, and Mason himself, while refusing to stay in the hospital, does agree to go with his friends, who have offered to drive him to his parents' home. Given these circumstances there is good reason not to override Mason's refusal to stay in the hospital. He should be allowed to go with his friends (provided they can control him). So, in general, a sufficient degree of irrationality provides a strong reason, but not necessarily a justification, for overriding a person's right to consent.

But what counts as a suffcent degree of irrationality? How irrational does a person have to be for us to have a strong reason to override his right to consent? Here we must explain what we mean when we call a person irrational.

Irrationality. Basically, a person is irrational if the ways in which he gains, stores, and uses information deviate—in an unproductive way— from the ways in which people normally gain, store, and use information.[12] To understand this claim, and especially to understand the terms *unproductive* and *normally,* let us look at an example in which a person gains, stores, and uses information in the normal ways—driving a car. To drive a car successfully you have to gain—by your perceptions— information about the road you are on, about the speed and position of your car, and about the speed and position of other cars. You use this information to determine what to do when driving. For example, if the road curves to the left, your perception of this must lead you to turn to the left a certain degree—provided you want to avoid an accident.

In general, at any given moment of our waking life we are gaining information by our perceptions. We also have a great deal of information stored in the form of our beliefs and memories. And we use this information in guiding our actions, in reasoning our way to new conclusions and ideas, and in making decisions. To gain, store, and use information is to process it. Now, the basic point we want to make is this. As the driving-the-car example illustrates, a normal human being has the capacity to process information in specific ways that are generally successful in getting him what he wants. In part this is the definition of what it is to be a normal human being. We will not try to say what these particular ways of processing information are; that is a task for psychology. We will for convenience simply call them the normal ways.

Nobody always processes information in the normal ways; in fact, we all deviate frequently from the normal ways because of fatigue, fear, inattention, or depression. These factors often affect our thinking, perceiving, and reasoning, and often affect it for the worse. So, what does *normal* refer to here? It refers to the ways in which we would process information if no factors—such as inattention—interfered. We have a certain capacity to process information. We do not always perform up to capacity; but if we are normal the capacity exists.

Mason's case illustrates these points well. Mason is irrational because he does not—and by and large cannot—process information in the normal ways, and because the ways in which he does handle information are unproductive—that is, they are not successful in getting him what he wants. We may suppose that Mason wants continued life as a physically healthy human being. However, his belief that he possesses a death-ray could easily lead to reckless aggressive actions which would endanger his health and life. He has already assaulted the police officers who brought him to the hospital. Generally, Mason has an ideal self-image, an image which may include such things as being a successful student, but Mason's ways of processing information are not conducive to realizing this image. Since Mason (like all of us) will not be happy unless he realizes at least some aspects of his ideal self-image, we should not regard his ways of processing information as successful unless they are conducive to realizing that self-image—unless, that is, they effectively promote his self-realization.[13] In general our position will be that *ways of processing information are successful in getting a person what he wants if and only if they lead him to act in a way that effectively promotes his self-realization.*

If Mason's unusual ways of handling information were successful in getting him what he wants, we would not regard him as irrational; we might regard him as strange. Or if he was significantly better at getting what he wants than the average person, we might regard him as very lucky, or highly intelligent, or both. In general, however, we think we ought to process information in the normal ways; we regard lapses of memory and inattention as things which ought not to happen—at least in those cases in which we are attempting to deal effectively with our environment. And our attitude makes sense. Unless we have a good reason to put another's concerns before our own, we should use the most effective means at our disposal to get what we want. It is irrational not to do so. Now, for most of us anyway, the best means at our disposal are the normal ways of processing information. When we judge a person like Mason against this standard, we regard him as irrational, and it is the extreme degree of his irrationality that gives us a strong reason to override his right to consent.

Degrees of irrationality. This brings us back to the question of what counts as a sufficient degree of irrationality. How irrational does a person have to be for us to have a strong reason to override his right to consent? The first point to note is that *the degree of irrationality is measured by the person's ability to function in his environment— to be successful in getting what he wants.* When a person is a danger to himself or others, the degree is clearly extreme and we have a good reason to override the person's right to consent. But what should we do when the degree of irrationality is less than this? There is no single answer to this question. Degrees of irrationality form a continuum.

At one end we have the occasional, minor departures from the normal ways of processing information which we all exhibit, departures which are so common and so minor they hardly deserve to be called irrational. They are just the result of fatigue, inattention, anxiety, or carelessness. But as the frequency or degree of deviation increases the label of irrationality becomes more and more appropriate. A severe depression (like Miller's), for example, can result in prolonged and extreme irrationality as the person lapses into a state of inattention and apathy and refuses to deal with his environment.

Degrees of irrationality shade into one another, and there is no way to draw a sharp line across this continuum and divide it neatly in two so that on one side of the line we have a strong reason to override the right to consent while on the other side we do not. Each case must be considered separately. We have seen that a degree of irrationality always gives us some reason to override the right to consent, and the strength of the reason increases as the degree of irrationality increases, but in each case we must weigh the reasons for and against violating the right to consent. This is how things stand from a moral point of view.

From a moral point of view irrationality is a constant factor in those situations in which we are considering overriding the right to consent. Are there any other constant factors that should always be considered in such situations? The answer, I think, is that there are two factors: consent and danger. In the next section we will identify and explain these factors, and after doing so we will be able to formulate a principle of proxy consent which applies to mental patients. If we decide to override the consent of a mentally disturbed person, this certainly does not mean we can just do as we please with him; he is still a person with all of a person's rights. What should we do? And what shouldn't we do? The principle of proxy consent we will develop is aimed at answering these questions.

3. A principle of proxy consent

Irrationality, consent, and danger are the three constant factors we should always consider when faced with the question of whether to override a mentally disturbed person's right to consent. We can clarify and illustrate the role these factors play by returning to the two examples of consent we considered in section 1—Miller's case and the dog phobia case. Violations of the right to consent occur in each, and we want to see how these violations can be justified.

In Miller's case—the attempted suicide—we saw that Miller's right to consent was overridden twice—once by the doctor who saved his life and once by the psychiatrist who talked to him afterwards. Let us examine the second violation, the one by the psychiatrist.

The psychiatrist who sees Miller after his suicide attempt overrides Miller's right to give or withhold free and informed consent by deliberately manipulating Miller into opting for short-term therapy. He influences Miller's decision to such a degree that the decision cannot be regarded as free. What justifies this? To answer this question we need to consider the three factors of irrationality, danger, and consent. The justification of the psychiatrist's actions will turn out to be rather lengthy, but it is worth going into this case in detail to illustrate the complex and subtle nature of the issue of consent in psychiatry and psychotherapy.

Irrationality. There are two claims to consider: First, Miller's depression makes him irrational; second, this irrationality is an essential factor in justifying the psychiatrist's violation of Miller's right to consent. As to the first claim, a person is irrational provided that the ways in which he processes information deviate in an unproductive way from the ways in which people normally process information. Miller's depression makes him irrational because it makes him deviate from the normal ways of processing information and because this deviation is unproductive—that is, it works against Miller's getting what he wants.

To see just how Miller deviates, the first point we should note is that Miller's depression leads him to accept false information about himself—information he would not accept if he were processing information in the normal ways. This false information is that he no longer wants to live when, in fact, the opposite is true. He accepts this information because his depression distorts his perception of his own desires. His grief at his wife's death leads to the impulse not to live any longer, and because of his severe depression he interprets this impulse to be what he really wants.

Now, if Miller were processing information in the normal ways, he would not make this mistake, for then he would distinguish between his impulses and what he really wants. The ability to distinguish between impulses and what you really want is characteristic of processing information in the normal ways. For example, suppose you have a sudden impulse to drink a can of yellow paint. One reason you do not give into this impulse is that you recognize it is incompatible with other things you really want, such as to stay healthy, and it would be a serious deviation from the normal ways of processing information to regard this impulse as something you really want. Miller does deviate in this way when he interprets his impulse not to live any longer as something he really wants. And this deviation is obviously unproductive since it leads to a suicide attempt when what Miller really wants is to continue to live.

So, Miller is irrational, and it is this irrationality which is essential to justifying the psychiatrist's violation of his right to consent. If Miller were not irrational, what reason could we give for overriding his right to consent? None. However, as we saw in the last section, a degree of irrationality always provides us with some reason to override the right to consent, and the greater the degree of irrationality, the stronger the reason. In Miller's case the degree of irrationality is certainly substantial since it leads to a suicide attempt when Miller really wants to live.[14] Is it a sufficient degree of irrationality to justify overriding Miller's right to consent? To answer this question we need to turn to the factors of danger and consent.

Danger. Even after his suicide attempt Miller is still a danger to himself. Although he really wants to live he is still depressed, and his depression is still distorting his perceptions of his own desires so that he thinks he does not want to live. What role does the factor of danger play in justifying what the psychiatrist does? In answering this question it is helpful to contrast the psychiatrist's violation of Miller's right to consent with the doctor's violation of that right.

For the doctor, danger plus Miller's irrationality are enough to justify the violation of Miller's right to consent—the violation involved in saving Miller's life. For the doctor the alternatives are clear. Save Miller's life or let him die, and since Miller really wants to live saving his life is obviously best. (The doctor naturally and justifiably assumes Miller really wants to live since this is what the vast majority of people really want.) It is the alternative which best fits in with Miller's plans and projects. Miller himself does not think so, but the combination of danger and irrationality justify overriding his right to consent in this situation.

In contrast with the doctor, the situation the psychiatrist faces is not so clear cut. The psychiatrist is convinced that short-term therapy would be best for Miller, but the alternatives are not either getting Miller to choose short-term therapy or letting Miller die, for there are two other possibilities. Perhaps Miller might recover from his depression on his own, or perhaps he might eventually decide on his own in favor of therapy. Do the factors of danger and irrationality justify the psychiatrist in closing off these possibilities by manipulating Miller into opting for short-term therapy? These factors might be sufficient to justify this. The crucial issue is the likelihood of either of the two possibilities. The more unlikely it is that Miller will pull out of the depression on his own or opt for therapy on his own, the stronger the psychiatrist's case for manipulating him into short-term therapy. Contrast Miller's case with

Mason's case, which we discussed in the last section. Mason was extremely irrational—for example, believing he was communicating by mental telepathy with beings from outer space—and it was highly unlikely that Mason would recover on his own before he harmed himself or someone else. Miller's case is not as clear since he certainly might pull out of his depression by himself.

The general situation is this. The degree of irrationality needed to justify overriding a person's right to consent decreases as the danger of the person to himself or others increases. A person who is a danger to himself or others is likely to interfere with either his or someone else's pursuit of self-realization. So, danger is always a factor that should be considered. But in Miller's case it is not clear that the combination of this factor with Miller's irrationality justifies the psychiatrist's overriding his right to consent because of the possibility that Miller could pull out of his depression on his own.

In spite of this unclarity, however, the psychiatrist is justified in overriding Miller's right to consent. To see why, we need to examine the factor of consent.

Consent. Miller does give consent to talking with the psychiatrist. The psychiatrist walks in, says who he is, and asks to talk. Miller could always refuse, but in our example he does not. Instead, he agrees to talk. Now, we can assume Miller knows that the psychiatrist may try to influence him and that he may try to do so by concealed manipulation. Many people know this is the nature of psychiatric interviews and therapy sessions, and we will assume Miller is one of them. So, by consenting to talk, Miller does give his consent to some concealed manipulation. In general, *to consent to psychotherapy is to consent to concealed manipulation—to some extent.* In those cases in which a person does not realize this is the nature of psychotherapy, his giving or withholding of consent will not be informed unless he is presented with the information that psychotherapy may involve concealed manipulation to some extent.

Of course, the crucial phrase here is "to some extent." In Miller's case, for example, does the fact that he has consented to some possible manipulation justify the psychiatrist's manipulating Miller into short-term therapy? Even given Miller's consent to talking with the psychiatrist, this manipulation is still a violation of his right to consent since his decision in favor of short-term therapy is not free. Does Miller's consent to talking with the therapist justify manipulation to this extent?

Let us review the situation. The factors of irrationality and danger give us a reason to override Miller's right to consent. The fact that Miller has consented to some concealed manipulation strengthens this reason, for Miller has given his consent to letting the psychiatrist try to influence him. *This is certainly enough to justify the psychiatrist in doing something about Miller's suicidal depression; it is enough to justify some concealed manipulation by the psychiatrist.* The important point is that the combination of consent, irrationality, and danger may justify overriding the right to consent even when the combination of just irrationality and danger does not or does not clearly do so. This is what happens in Miller's case; the addition of the factor of consent justifies the psychiatrist in doing something. But exactly what should he do? What he does is manipulate Miller into opting for short-term therapy. Why is that what he should do?

Ideally the psychiatrist should accomplish his goal of bringing Miller out of his suicidal depression while interfering as little as possible in Miller's life. This is the ideal because Miller (like everyone) has the right to self-determination. So, each of us has a reason (of a special sort)[15] not to interfere with Miller's pursuit of those plans and projects he believes will lead to his self-realization. Suppose we had a choice between two forms of concealed manipulation—both of which had an equal chance of getting Miller out of his depression. Given that Miller has the right to self-determination, we should choose the form of manipulation which interferes least with Miller's pursuit of his plans and projects. Of course, if one form of manipulation were more effective than the other, we would have to weigh the degree of effectiveness against the degree of interference. In general, we want to maximize the effectiveness of the treatment while minimizing the degree of interference. The best compromise between these two goals is what we should choose. Now, manipulating Miller into short-term therapy is justified if it is the best compromise between these two goals. But is it the best compromise?

Ordinarily we would allow Miller himself to answer a question like this, but we have already justified taking the decision out of Miller's hands and putting it in the hands of the psychiatrist. It is essentially Miller's irrationality—combined with the factors of danger and consent—which disqualifies him as the judge of what best fits in with his plans, while the psychiatrist's manipulative knowledge and skill qualifies him as a judge about what will be effective in dealing with Miller's depression. Still, we do not want to give the psychiatrist a free hand in using his knowledge and skill. We want him to make the best compromise between the effectiveness of treatment and the degree of interference in Miller's life.

There is a rule for making such compromises. The rule is this: the psychiatrist should make the choice which he has good reason to think Miller himself would make if Miller were rational and possessed the information about depression and its treatment which the psychiatrist possesses. What the rule does is combine the two things we want combined—Miller's plans and the psychiatrist's skill and knowledge. The choice the psychiatrist makes will be responsive to Miller's plans and projects because it will be the choice the psychiatrist thinks Miller himself would make if he were rational. This protects Miller's personal freedom and his right to self-determination. The psychiatrist's choice will also be responsive to the psychiatrist's expert knowledge and skill because it will be the choice the psychiatrist thinks Miller would make if he were rational *and* possessed the information about depression and its treatment which the psychiatrist possesses. This helps ensure that an effective treatment will be chosen.

When we apply this rule to Miller's case manipulation into short-term therapy turns out to be what the psychiatrist should choose. To apply the rule we should imagine Miller outside his situation, so to speak, directing the scene in which he plays the role of the patient treated by the psychiatrist. Our claim is that Miller would direct the psychiatrist to manipulate him into short-term therapy—provided that Miller was rational and possessed the relevant information. Miller would do this because if he were rational he would realize he really wants to live, and so he would want to recover. And if he possessed the psychiatrist's information about depression and its treatment, he would realize that short-term therapy is an effective way of dealing with his depression and also involves only a minimal interference with his plans and projects. The interference is minimal for several reasons. To begin with, short-term therapy is just that—short-term. In addition, the therapy has the limited and definite goal of getting Miller out of his depression; it does not aim at altering his personality. Also, Miller can choose his therapist and he can stop therapy whenever he wants. So, all things considered, there is good reason to think that Miller would choose short-term therapy if he were rational and possessed the relevant information.

It follows, then, that the psychiatrist is justified in manipulating Miller into opting for short-term therapy. We can now generalize from our justification of this particular instance of manipulation to obtain a general principle of proxy consent which covers cases like Miller's. To see how to do this, consider the following abstraction of Miller's case. There are two people involved—x (the psychiatrist) and y (Miller). What happens is that x overrides y's right to consent by manipulating y in a certain way M (manipulating Miller into short-term therapy). Some form of manipulation is justified by the three factors of irrationality, danger, and consent. These factors justify doing something to achieve a certain therapeutic goal G (getting Miller out of his depression). Manipulation in way M in order to achieve G is justified by the rule that x (the psychiatrist) should make the choice he has good reason to think y (Miller) would freely consent to if y were rational and possessed x's information about M and G. So, x is justified in making a decision for y; in effect, x gives proxy consent for y to M in order to achieve G. Of course, x would not be justified here if his information about M did not represent a well-informed expert opinion about M (manipulation into short-term therapy) and G (curing depression). It is partly the psychiatrist's expert knowledge that makes him qualified to decide for Miller.

We can abstract the following principle of proxy consent from the preceding description:[16]

(P3) x should override y's right to consent in manipulating y in way M in order to achieve a therapeutic goal G if and only if x has good reason to think y would freely consent to manipulation in way M in order to achieve G if y were rational and possessed x's information about M and G, and x's information about M and G represents a well-informed opinion.

(P3) applies in those cases in which some combination of the factors of irrationality, danger, and consent already justify doing something in order to achieve the therapeutic goal G. (P3) is intended as a guideline to help us choose a morally acceptable treatment from a set of reasonable medical alternatives.

There are two practical problems which arise in applying (P3). The first is determining when a person is irrational; the second, determining what counts as well-informed opinion. Both these problems are well illustrated by the case in which the parents come to the therapist because of their son's dog phobia (section 1, example 2).

Let us take the irrationality problem first. We said that a person is irrational if he deviates unproductively from the normal ways of processing information. But we did not say what the normal ways are. How can we identify the deviations of irrationality if we have not identified the normal ways of processing information? The dog phobia case suggests a solution to this problem. Recall that the therapist treats the parents for their marital problem and that he does so without their consent. The parents must be irrational to some degree if this is to be justified.[17] But is it clear that the parents are irrational? Their behavior is not openly bizarre like Mason's—who was found running naked down a city street. Nor is it obviously self-destructive like Miller's attempted suicide. If they are irrational the manifestation is subtle. Can we spot a subtle manifestation of irrationality without a clear idea of what counts as a normal way of processing information?

The answer is *yes*, to some extent, because we do have a fairly good idea of what we expect normal people to be able to do. It is not a precise idea, but it is not useless either. Consider the parents in our example. They have—unconsciously perhaps—let a situation develop in which they relate to each other only through their son, and this situation is seriously harming their child and making them unhappy as well. The situation is right before their eyes, yet they fail to consciously recognize and deal with it. *We would expect a person who was gaining information about the world in normal ways to recognize it, but the parents do not.* Therefore, they are irrational to some degree. Since they are, the therapist might be justified in overriding their right to consent. The question is: Do the factors of irrationality, consent, and danger justify doing so? We will leave this question unanswered (you may work out an answer on your own).

Instead, we will turn to the second practical problem: determining what counts as a well-informed opinion. A well-informed opinion is one based on accurate and complete information. The practical problem is that it is not clear in psychiatry what counts as accuracy and completeness, for there is considerable disagreement, even among experts, both about the diagnosis of mental disorders and about what treatments are most effective. In the dog phobia case the therapeutic approach is aimed at solving a specific problem; it is not intended to produce insight or understanding in the patient but rather to manipulate him in such a way that the problem disappears. Not every therapist shares this conception of the aims of psychotherapy.

Faced with disagreement among even the experts, how should we apply (P3) in practice? What we should do is try to ensure that our information is as accurate and complete as possible. The situation is hardly hopeless. There is a considerable body of clinical knowledge about how to diagnose and treat mental patients. You can find such data summarized in handbooks and manuals.[18]

The practical difficulties of determining what counts as a well-informed opinion about diagnosis and treatment are connected with the problem of defining mental disorders, for the former will certainly depend in part on our definitions.

4. The problem of definition

We noted at the beginning of this chapter that we tend to regard a mental disorder as evidence that we may be justified in overriding the person's right to consent. The problem of definition of mental disorder is central to this issue. It is also worth examining for its own sake. For when we define a mental disorder we are saying that people who fit the definition are unhealthy, and that they are unhealthy because of the way in which they think, feel, and act. Can we justify regarding these people as unhealthy? Or are we just arbitrarily imposing our views about how to live on those people who fit our definitions of mental disorders?

Consider the case of Fanny, a woman in her early twenties. Fanny is the sort of person whom psychiatrists would class as a borderline personality; in particular, one who exhibits what is known as rejection-sensitive dysphoria, a tendency to become desperate and unhappy when disapproved of or rejected. Such people are by and large women.[19] In the *Manual of Psychiatric Therapeutics*, the general state of such a woman is described as

an extremely brittle, shallow mood ranging from giddy elation to desperate unhappiness and markedly responsive to external sources of admiration and approval. Such a patient may appear hopelessly bereft when a love affair terminates, but upon meeting a new attentive man, she may feel perfectly fine and even slightly elated within a few days. Similarly, failure to win high praise for their work may devastate them, but the trauma is quickly forgotten if this gap if filled by commendation for another project. This emotionality markedly affects their judgment. When euphoric, they minimize and deny shortcomings of a situation or personal relationship, idealizing all achievements and love objects. But when they are at the opposite emotional pole, feelings of desperation disproportionate to the actual circumstances are expressed.[20]

Fanny fits this description perfectly. She also has the other traits commonly associated with this sort of borderline personality. She is "seductive, manipulative, exploitive, sexually provocative, and emotional and illogical,"[21] and in sexual relationships she is "possessive, grasping, demanding, romantic."[22] She views people as essentially ways to adjust her mood; Fanny virtually never appreciates others for what they are in themselves and does not really understand the complexities of other people.

What makes this a mental disorder? Most of us have known women at least somewhat like Fanny, for our society promotes such behavior in women. As the *Manual of Psychiatric Therapeutics* says:

In our society, as probably in most others, a primary goal in the life of many women is to attract and retain a supporting male figure. . . . Among the social tactics available to women, and approved of as peculiarly feminine, are exhibitionistic, seductive displays of their charms. Women with a normal range of emotional response utilize a wide variety of exhibitionistic and seductive social tactics with discretion and accuracy. The female hysteriod dysphoric patient is a caricature of femininity because her disorder drives her to attempt to repair her dysphoria by exaggerating the social, seductive, exhibitionistic tactics allowable to women in our society. It is the driven quality and repetitiousness of behavior that indicates the underlying affective disorder.[23]

We can agree with the description of the "social tactics" available to women in our society. That much seems true, and it explains why most of us have encountered women at least somewhat like Fanny.

But does "the driven quality and repetitiousness of behavior" indicate a mental disorder ("the underlying affective disorder")? Why isn't Fanny just an extreme example of the sort of behavior which some women exhibit in our society? *What makes her sick as opposed to just extreme?* Unless we can answer this question, we are wrong to regard Fanny as mentally disordered. Indeed, radical feminists who reject the notion of femininity described in the last passage quoted might accuse us of just such a mistake. They might claim that, not only does society mold women into a pattern which—from the point of view of radical feminism—is degrading, but it also punishes women like Fanny who exhibit this pattern to an extreme degree. It punishes them by categorizing them as mentally ill, as unhealthy and in need of treatment, and this categorization endangers their rights since they may be discriminated against on the basis of it. Can we answer these charges? Or are they correct?

Using Fanny as an example, the key to the answer is the fact that Fanny's changes in mood—her "emotionality"—affect her ability to think and judge. There are two basic points to be made. First, Fanny's emotionality makes her irrational to a high degree. And second, this high degree of irrationality is what is crucial to categorizing her as mentally ill. We will consider each claim in turn.

Fanny's emotionality makes her irrational provided that it makes her deviate unproductively from the normal ways of processing information. Now, it certainly makes her deviate. The strength and instability of her moods "markedly affects" her judgment so that she thinks her situation is either much better or much worse than it is. In addition, this deviation is not an aberration but a constant feature of her life. But is the deviation unproductive—that is, does it stand in the way of Fanny's getting what she wants?

To answer this question we need a more detailed description of Fanny's case, so let us imagine how she might appear to a therapist who treats her. Her therapist might describe her as follows:

This 22-year-old female was a school dropout, sometimes alcoholic, occasionally a drug user, promiscuous, and had one illegitimate pregnancy and abortion. Her psychotherapeutic sessions have been filled with accounts of vacillation between Joe and Larry, always breaking up with one or the other. No evidence of any affectionate relationship was ever found, not even to a dog she bought and permitted to die. . . .[24]

In one session Fanny described her relation with Larry and Joe; her therapist is the "I" of the following passage.

She said, "I'm so disgusted, I just feel that nobody cares." I asked if that included Joe and Larry. She said, "Yes." I said, "It seems like you would like to have closeness and concern and yet, when it is within your grasp, there is something about it that seems to make you flee from it." After a long silence she said, "Yeah, I know that's true. I can see that now. But what do I do about it?" I asked her what there was about the closeness that forced her to break it off. She said, "Well, when you get into a relationship like that, you get trapped. At first it's fine. But then you start getting into a pattern. You have to do what the other one wants you to do. . . . It's like when I sleep with a boy for a few months. At first it's exciting and fun. And, then after a while, I just have to keep going. Not 'cause I want to any more. Then I want to be free. I want to get out of the relationship, and I don't know how to do it. So then I start creating little incidents so that the other one will have to break up with me. I want my freedom then, but then, when I have my freedom I just feel lonely again."[25]

The point is that Fanny is unable to form any lasting, satisfying relationships, and this inability is directly related to the ways in which her moods affect her judgment. This inability to form lasting, satisfying relationships also makes Fanny basically an extremely unhappy woman, so her deviation from the normal ways of processing information must definitely be counted as unproductive.

So, Fanny is irrational, and in fact she is irrational to a high degree since her irrationality makes her quite unhappy.[26] Now, it is her high degree of irrationality which is crucial to justifying our regarding her as mentally ill. As we argued earlier, to be unhealthy is to deviate from normal ways of functioning in an unproductive way,[27] and we have just seen that Fanny deviates from the normal ways of processing information and that this deviation is unproductive. Consequently, she is unhealthy—mentally unhealthy because her deviation takes the form of irrationality. Indeed, if Fanny were not irrational, we would be wrong to regard her as mentally ill. Then she would just be an extreme case of a woman who exploits the "social tactics" described earlier, and the extreme, the bizarre, and the unusual are not necessarily unhealthy. If Fanny was merely extreme and we classified her as mentally ill, we would have no defense to the radical feminist charge that we were simply punishing her for being an extreme version of what society makes some women become. It is only irrationality that allows us to draw the distinction between the extreme and the unusual on one side and the mentally ill on the other.

In general, then, a definition of a mental disorder is justified only if we can show that people who fit the definition are irrational to a relatively high degree. Now, there is no way to fix precisely what counts as a relatively high degree of irrationality. As we noted in section 2, we all frequently depart from the normal ways of processing information. How great and frequent do these deviations have to be to raise the issue of mental illness? I see no general answer to this question. The more irrationality we require before we count a person as mentally ill, the more tolerant we will be of the extreme, the bizarre, and the unusual. The less irrationality we require, the greater the number of people who will be included under our definitions, and—perhaps—the greater the number of people who will have their problems identified and helped by therapy. What we want to do here is compromise between tolerating the extreme and the unusual and constructing clinically useful definitions.

Irrationality provides just one requirement of the definition of a mental disorder. We will not provide a complete explanation of what counts as a definition of a mental disorder.[27] A complete theory would have to consider such questions as can a mental disorder be defined by simply citing a certain collection of symptoms? Or must the definition describe a specific underlying sequence of mental or physical causes which produce the symptoms? These are issues in the philosophy of science, and we will leave them unanswered.

To summarize, we have singled out the irrationality requirement to demonstrate that a definition of a mental disorder is justified only if a sufficient degree of irrationality is exhibited by people who fit the definition. It is essential to insist on this point in order to safeguard the rights of those people who are simply strange, extreme, or peculiar in some way. It is also essential in order to explain why a person who fits the definition of a mental disorder is unhealthy. What makes the person count as unhealthy is the unproductive deviation from the normal ways of processing information. In addition, the requirement of irrationality explains why we regard a mental disorder as evidence that we may be justified in overriding that person's right to consent. As we saw in section 2, a sufficient degree of irrationality gives us a strong reason to override a person's right to consent. Finally, it is essential to note the role of irrationality in definitions of mental disorders in order to prepare for the discussion of our final topic, the problem of deviance.

5. Deviance: what should be done?

Deviant people are individuals who are socially maladjusted or psychologically abnormal. The question we want to consider is: Should we use therapy, drugs, and psychosurgery to control the behavior of such people—even when they withhold consent to these means of control? Let us first consider a number of examples in order to see the extent and complexity of the problem of deviance.

First example: compulsory sterilization.   Sarah is a mentally retarded eighteen-year-old woman whose IQ is approximately 60. So, Sarah is a deviant, a psychologically abnormal person. She is also a warmhearted, kind young woman whose main goal at the moment is to have a baby of her own. Her mother, on the other hand, is convinced that Sarah could not adequately care for a child and thinks she should be sterilized. When she confronts her daughter with this idea, Sarah runs out of the house shouting back at her mother that she is going to her boyfriend's apartment and that no one will stop her from getting pregnant. Her boyfriend is also mentally retarded. Should Sarah's mother ask the court to order her daughter's sterilization?

Second example: a case of indecent exposure.   This is an actual case. In 1964 Charles H. Lomax was found to be mentally disordered[28] by the District Court of General Sessions of Washington, D.C. and was committed for an indefinite length of time to St. Elizabeth's Hospital in Washington, D.C. for psychiatric treatment. Lomax was originally charged with indecent exposure, and he had in fact exposed himself naked from the waist down to a woman passerby. Lomax had been convicted of indecent exposure sixteen years earlier, and under psychiatric examination he admitted to having exposed himself on other occasions. He also admitted that he often experiences a powerful impulse to expose himself, an impulse he has great difficulty in resisting. Should Lomax have been committed for an indeterminate period to a hospital for psychiatric treatment? Indecent exposure is a crime with a definite sentence, but since he was found to be mentally disordered, Lomax was not given this sentence but was sent off for psychiatric treatment instead.[30] This was done even though the psychiatrist testified that Lomax was not dangerous to others. Was this justified?

This example raises an important and difficult legal issue. Because Lomax is mentally disordered, we think that he should not be treated as a criminal—even though he has committed a crime. That makes sense. But it also raises the very difficult question of what the courts should do with him. This same issue comes up in our next example.

Third example: a case of assault. Dixon is a forty-five-year-old man who was committed to a psychiatric hospital for assaulting and maiming a woman. He invited her to his apartment and, once there, proceeded to tie her up and make small cuts in her with a knife. Then he let her go. After a year in the hospital Dixon petitions the court for his release, but the petition is denied when the hospital psychiatrist testifies Dixon would still be a danger to others if released. The psychiatrist testifies that Dixon has definite homosexual tendencies, and has in fact admitted to strong homosexual impulses. These impulses were often followed by acts of violence in an attempt to reassert his masculinity and reestablish his self-esteem. The psychiatrist insists this pattern of behavior will reappear if Dixon is released.[31] What should be done with Dixon? And who should decide?

Fourth example: "vent-man". This is the example of deviance we gave in section 1—the example of Kelly, the vagrant known as "vent-man" because of his habit of sleeping on a steam vent in cold weather.[32] Kelly is a basically harmless psychotic whose behavior is, however, occasionally disruptive; for he sometimes blocks traffic and sometimes shouts insults at passersby. The police and the psychiatric staff of the local hospital cooperate to control Kelly's behavior. When he is too disruptive the police pick him up and bring him to the hospital where his disruptive behavior can be controlled by drugs. The aim of the drug therapy is just to control and not to cure since it is highly unlikely that a well-established psychosis like Kelly's will respond to such treatment. Are we justified in controlling Kelly's behavior in this way? And, if so, would we be justified in using similar means to control the behavior of Dixon in the previous example?

As these four examples illustrate, a wide variety of issues and cases are included under the problem of deviance. We can systematize this variety by distinguishing between different types of deviant individuals, for to know how to deal with deviance we need to know what we are dealing with. What we want to know is when are we justified in over-riding the right to consent of a deviant person in order to force him to undergo some form of psychiatric treatment? We also want to focus on the question of how the courts should handle deviant individuals who commit crimes.

The rational and the irrational. A deviant person is one who is socially maladjusted or psychologically abnormal, but this does not mean that deviant people are always mentally disordered. In fact, a deviant individual need not even be irrational. For example, a man who lives alone without friends, and who has no desire to make friends, is not necessarily irrational although he is certainly deviant since he is definitely abnormal psychologically. Some deviant people, however, are deviant at least in part because they are irrational,[33] because they deviate unproductively from the normal ways of processing information. Sarah, in our preceding example is deviant because of her irrationality—or, more precisely, because of her mental retardation. This counts as an example of deviance because of irrationality since mental retardation is an unproductive deviation from the normal ways of processing information.

In general, we should distinguish between those deviant people who are deviant because they are irrational and those who are deviant but not irrational.[34] The distinction is important because there is no special moral or legal problem about people who are deviant but not irrational. Like any other person a deviant individual has the right to self-determination, and deviance alone without irrationality provides no ground for overriding this right by interfering with the deviant person's conduct of his life. The right to self-determination protects the deviant—the strange, the extreme, the bizarre—up to the point of irrationality. However, with those who are deviant because they are irrational, the factor of irrationality provides us with some reason for overriding such persons' right to consent. The question is when and how—if ever—we should do so. First, we need to distinguish between those deviant people who are dangerous and those who are not.

Dangerous or not dangerous. Among those who are deviant because they are irrational, some are dangerous and some are not. There is a range of cases here as the examples we gave earlier illustrate. For instance, consider Dixon who is clearly a danger to others since he commits acts of violence to restore his threatened sense of masculinity. At the other extreme Kelly, the vent-man, is basically harmless and would be completely harmless if he did not block traffic and shout at passersby. Lomax, on the other hand, falls in between Dixon and Kelly. His behavior is offensive and could conceivably be psychologically harmful to others. Also, it might be dangerous to him—for example, if he were severely beaten by someone who was outraged by one of his acts of indecent exposure. Finally, Sarah, is an unclear case. Her mental retardation might make her a danger to herself and also to any child she may bear, but it also might not.

The distinction between irrational deviants[35] who are dangerous and those who are not is important mainly from a legal point of view. In those cases in which an irrational deviant person completely withholds consent to psychiatric treatment, we should make it legal to override his right to consent only if the person is a danger to himself or others. To see why, we should contrast the legal with the moral situation. As we saw in section 2, a sufficient degree of irrationality may—even without the factor of danger—morally justify overriding a person's right to consent. So, morally speaking, we are justified in overriding a deviant person's right to consent when there is sufficient degree of irrationality. Of course, the factors of danger and consent may also play a role in justifying this.

Now, why should we create a difference between what is required for a legal, as opposed to a moral, justification? The reason is that the requirements for a legal justification must be clear and definite in order to prevent abuse through intentional or unintentional misinterpretation and misapplication. This is especially important in framing the legal requirements for overriding the right to consent of a deviant individual, for we want to safeguard the rights of deviants who are not irrational. The moral requirement of a sufficient degree of irrationality is not clear and definite enough for a legal requirement—for the simple reason that the moral requirement does not specify what counts as a sufficient degree. We have seen that there is no way to draw a line across the continuum of irrationality and divide it so that on one side we have a strong moral reason to override the right to consent while on the other side we do not. Legally speaking, however, we should draw a sharp line across the continuum of irrationality since we need a clear and definite criterion for overriding the right to consent of an irrational deviant person by forcing him to undergo psychiatric treatment.

The criterion should be danger to oneself or others. More precisely, *overriding the right to consent of a deviant person who is deviant because he is irrational should be legal only in those cases in which the person is a danger to himself or others.* This is the only way to draw a line across the continuum of irrationality which is sufficiently clear and definite to serve as a legal criterion. We will not defend this claim;[36] instead, we will examine the issue of what counts as danger to oneself or others.

Like degrees of irrationality, degrees of danger form a continuum ranging from cases like Kelly's to cases like Dixon's. So, if we want a clear and definite legal requirement for overriding the right to consent of an irrational deviant individual, we need to draw a sharp line across this continuum also. How are we to do it? I suggest that an irrational deviant is a clear and definite danger to himself or others provided that one of the following two conditions holds: Either (1) the person has recently committed a harmful (or potentially harmful) act toward himself or another; or (2) there is strong evidence that he might commit such an act in the near future.

If we were actually constructing a legal requirement, we would have to explain exactly what "recently" and "harmful" mean in (1), and what "strong evidence" and "near future" mean in (2). Since legal issues are not our main concern, we will only consider here the practical difficulties of applying our suggested legal requirement. Requirements more or less like ours are common,[37] so it is worth considering these difficulties even though we have not argued for our requirement's correctness.

The position we have reached is that the right to consent of a deviant person may be overridden by forcing him to undergo psychiatric treatment provided that the person is deviant because he is irrational and is also a clear and definite danger to himself or others. The practical difficulties of this position can be seen by considering the four examples with which we began this section.

First example. Can we override the right to consent of Sarah, the mentally retarded girl, by forcing her to be sterilized? She is an irrational deviant individual, but is she a clear and definite danger to herself or others? She has not committed a harmful or potentially harmful act toward herself or others; so, if she is to be regarded as a clear and definite danger to herself or others there must be strong evidence that she will commit such an act in the near future. Is there such evidence? The only act she will commit in the near future which might count as harmful or potentially harmful to herself or others is getting pregnant and giving birth. This might be psychologically and physically dangerous both to her and her child if she proves unable to care for herself and her child. However, it is far from obvious that she will be unable to care for herself and her child. With an IQ of 60 she is not so severely retarded that she is obviously incapable of this. To determine her ability to care for a child we would have to consider the details of the particular case.

There is an argument that Sarah's having a child constitutes a danger to others; there is a chance that Sarah's child will be mentally retarded, for there is a statistically significant correlation between mental retardation in parents and mental retardation in their offspring.[38] Now, it might be harmful to others to bring a mentally retarded child into existence. We live in a world in which the resources available to us are insufficient to satisfy the wants of all people. A mentally retarded person is a potential drain on our scarce economic and medical resources since such a person may require special care. So, by being a drain on our resources the mentally retarded person might—by his very existence—harm others. Whether this is so has to be settled by a detailed examination of the economic and social facts.

The question of whether we should override Sarah's right to consent is unclear because of the complex psychological, economic, and social factors involved. One consequence of our proposed legal requirement is that, in applying it, we are forced to consider such factors. The fair administration of justice in this area requires a thorough knowledge of the complex interplay of psychological, economic, and social facts and issues.

Second example. What should have been done with Charles H. Lomax, the man who committed an act of indecent exposure? He was in fact committed indefinitely for psychiatric treatment. Was this right? Let us grant that Lomax is an irrational deviant. The question is whether he is a clear and definite danger to others. He has committed an act of indecent exposure and may do so again. If Lomax is to be regarded as a clear and definite danger, such acts must be regarded as harmful. This is an important consequence of our suggested legal requirement. We cannot ship people like Lomax off for psychiatric treatment simply because we find their behavior offensive. Is it harmful or at least potentially harmful? Perhaps it would be psychologically harmful to some people. This will depend on the community in which Lomax lives. It might also be psychologically damaging to Lomax; this will depend on Lomax—for example, on whether he feels guilt for exposing himself. It might also be physically dangerous to Lomax, for—depending again on the community—he might get severely beaten for exposing himself.

Again, we see how complex social and psychological factors enter into the application of our requirement. There are two further points which should be emphasized here. First, if we decide that Lomax is not a clear and definite danger, we should not override his right to consent by forcing him to undergo psychiatric treatment. But it is not clear what should be done with him. He could be convicted of indecent exposure and given the appropriate sentence, but is this what should be done? As we have noted, we tend to think that his mentally disordered state should keep him from being classified as a criminal. However, we cannot answer the question of what should be done with Lomax if he is found not to be a clear and definite danger because it is beyond the scope of this book.

The second point is if we do decide Lomax is a clear and definite danger, it does not follow that we should commit him to an indefinite period of psychiatric treatment. The overriding of the right to consent of an irrational deviant person must be adequately regulated by rules and procedures which protect the rights of the deviant person. *In particular, these rules and procedures should be designed to ensure that principle (P3) is followed,* for this is the principle of proxy consent which applies in cases of psychiatric patients. Now, it is not at all clear that these rules should allow commitment for an unspecified length of time since this can easily lead to abuses of a person's rights by encouraging lengthy periods of commitment.

Third example. Dixon's is a clear case. Dixon is obviously an irrational deviant who is a definite danger to others. Of course, our remarks about what to do with Lomax given that he is a danger also apply here. The essential difference between Lomax's case and Dixon's is Dixon's tendency to commit acts of physical violence toward others.

Fourth example. The case of Kelly, the vent-man, is at the opposite end of the spectrum from Dixon's. Kelly is also an irrational deviant. But is he a clear and definite danger? The most dangerous things he does are block traffic and shout at passersby, and he only does these things occasionally. Are these actions harmful? I doubt it. They may be inconvenient or offensive, but how could they be considered harmful? Now, if we decide they are not harmful, then our suggested legal requirement rules out forcing psychiatric treatment on Kelly. Of course, as with Lomax, the question of what should be done with Kelly still remains, for after all Kelly is sometimes a public nuisance. There are laws to deal with such cases, but should they be applied to Kelly? If Lomax is not a criminal, then surely Kelly is not either. What should be done?

This is one of the many questions about deviants we will leave unanswered. The problem of how to deal with deviants is extremely complex, and the aim of this section was just to survey some of the major issues.

6. Conclusion

Irrationality has been the central concept of this chapter. Now, it is frequently suggested that the question of whether a person is irrational or not is a subjective one, that it is merely a matter of personal opinion or social prejudice. Clarifying this issue will be an appropriate conclusion to this chapter.

Let us recall the definition of irrationality. A person is irrational provided that he deviates from the normal ways of processing information *and* provided that this deviation is unproductive—that is, unsuccessful in getting him what he wants. So, irrationality is a function of two factors: deviation and unproductiveness.

Whether someone deviates from the normal ways of processing information is clearly an objective question. Consider the example of Mason (section 2), who thinks he communicates by mental telepathy with beings from outer space—the Zircons. Now, Mason either processes information in the normal ways or he does not. And in Mason's case it is clear he does not. In general, the normal ways of processing information provide us with an objective standard against which we can assess the ways in which particular people process information.

But now consider the factor of unproductiveness. An unproductive deviation is one that is not successful in getting a person what he wants. Is the question of whether a person is successful in getting what he wants an objective one? In some cases it clearly is. For example, it is an objective question in the cases of Mason and Miller, the suicidal depressive (sections 1 and 3). These are extreme cases in which it is clear that many of their most important desires will go unsatisfied given the ways in which they deviate from the normal ways of processing information. But what about less extreme cases?

Recall that in section 2 we said that ways of processing information are successful in getting a person what he wants if and only if they lead him to act in ways that effectively promote his self-realization. Now, *effectively promoting self-realization* is a concept with vague boundaries. Just how effective does a person have to be to count as effectively promoting his self-realization? In borderline cases there will always be a subjective element in this decision. This means we should be especially careful in applying this notion in borderline cases; we want to compromise between tolerating the bizarre and the unusual and taking effective steps to alter the person's ways of acting in order to promote self-realization. To know how to make such compromises, we need a better understanding of the concepts of rationality and irrationality. It seems appropriate to end this chapter by recognizing this need. It is a reminder that our knowledge of the human mind is still very incomplete.

THEORETICAL FOUNDATIONS

We still have one theoretical issue to deal with. What is the justification of (P3)? (P3) says:

> x should override y's right to consent in manipulating y in way M to achieve a therapeutic goal G if and only if x has good reason to think y would freely consent to manipulation in way M in order to achieve G if y were rational and possessed x's information about M and G, and x's information about M and G represents a well-informed opinion.

In the typical case which we apply (P3), x is a therapist and y is his patient, and we defended (P3) earlier by pointing out that it combined two essentials—the patient's plans and projects and the therapist's knowledge and skill. The idea was that the choice the therapist makes in following (P3) will be responsive to the patient's plans and projects because it will be a choice the therapist has good reason to think the patient himself would make if he were rational. This protects the patient's right to self-determination. Now, the therapist's choice will also be responsive to the therapist's expert knowledge and skill since he will make the choice he has good reason to think the patient would make if he were rational and if he possessed the relevant information which the therapist in fact possesses. This helps ensure that the therapist will choose an effective treatment.

There is more to be said about how (P3) protects the patient's right to self-determination. It is true that the therapist's choice will be responsive to the patient's plans and projects because he will make a choice he has good reason to think the patient himself would make if the patient were rational. But the unanswered question is: Why should the choice be responsive to the patient's plans and projects *in just this way?* Why does *rationality* play the role of connecting the therapist's decision with the patient's plans and projects? The reason is that plans and rationality are connected in a certain way. A plan is general; it does not specify what to do in every possible contingency and circumstance. So, to carry out our plans, we must fill them out and fit them on to the circumstances which arise. Now, how do we fit plans on to the circumstances which arise? By gaining, storing, and using information in the normal ways—in short, by proceeding rationally. So, when the therapist makes his choice in accord with (P3), that choice is likely to correspond to the choice the patient himself would have made if he had not been mentally disordered.

FURTHER QUESTIONS

1. Was the therapist justified in overriding the patient's right to consent in the dog phobia case?

2. Is an attempted suicide always a sign of irrationality? If not, when is it not?

3. Should homosexuality be defined as a mental disorder?

4. What should be done with Kelly, the vent-man?

5. Are there different types of irrationality? If so, are these differences relevant to morality?

NOTES

1. See Chapter 1, section 5.
2. We faced similar problems in Chapters 1–3, but the two principles of proxy consent we used in those chapters are not appropriate to psychiatric cases.
3. See Chapter 2, note 20.
4. Legally, the doctor's action is justified. The law regards consent to medical treatment as implicit in any emergency situation.
5. Depending on Miller's exact state of mind, there are many ways in which this could be accomplished. Basically, the psychiatrist wants to create a context in which Miller will accept the suggestion of therapy.
6. This case is taken from Jay Haley, *Problem Solving Therapy* (San Francisco: Jossey-Bass, 1976), pp. 222–268. I should note here that Dr. Haley is aware of the ethical issues raised by his approach to therapy.
7. In the actual case the therapist did eventually discuss the marital problem and get consent to treating it.
8. *Diagnostic and Statistical Manual of Mental Disorders,* prepared by The Committee on Nomenclature and Statistics of the American Psychiatric Association, published by The American Psychiatric Association, Washington, D.C., 1968, p. 42.
9. See Nicholas N. Kittrie, *The Right to be Different* (Baltimore, Md.: Penguin, 1971), Chap. 1.
10. See Chapter 1, pp. 39–40.
11. Mason is also not free. He is the helpless victim of psychological forces he can neither identify nor control. However, this is not a feature of all mental disorders, so we leave it out of consideration here.

12. A deviation may be momentary or it may be long-term. We tend to classify people as irrational only when their deviation is more than just momentary. Also, we should distinguish this sense of *irrational* from our use of *rational choice* in Chapter 1. We are now talking about people—not choices—as being irrational or rational. Finally, we will not argue for our definition of irrationality. You can regard it as a stipulative definition if you like, although I think it is a correct explication of irrationality.

13. See Introduction, p. 11.

14. Recall that the degree of irrationality is measured by the person's ability to be successful in getting what he wants.

15. See Introduction, p. 12.

16. This is principle (P3) since we already have two other principles of proxy consent—(P1) and (P2). See Chapter 1, section 5.

17. We made this point in the discussion of Miller's case earlier in this section.

18. See, for example, Richard I. Shader, M.D. (ed.), *Manual of Psychiatric Therapeutics* (Boston: Little, Brown, 1975).

19. This fact is part of the reason for choosing the borderline personality as an example. I want to discuss the possible social implications of defining mental disorders.

20. *Manual of Psychiatric Therapeutics,* pp. 285–286.

21. *Manual,* p. 286.

22. *Manual,* p. 286.

23. *Manual,* p. 286.

24. Alfred M. Freedman, Harold I. Kaplan, and Benjamin J. Sadock (eds.), *Comprehensive Textbook of Psychiatry,* Vol. 1, 2nd ed. Williams and Wilkins, Baltimore 1975, p. 848.

25. *Comprehensive Textbook,* p. 848.

26. Recall that the degree is measured by her ability to be successful in getting what she wants.

27. For a discussion of these issues see Chapter 3 of Tom L. Beauchamp and LeRoy Walters, *Contemporary Issues in Bioethics* (Belmont, Calif.: Dickenson, 1978).

28. The legal classification used was *psychopath.*

29. This case is discussed in Kittrie, *The Right to be Different,* p. 171.

30. The court has the power to do this under the procedures for civil commitment.

31. Kittrie, *The Right to be Different* is an excellently documented, detailed, and insightful discussion of exactly this issue.

32. There is a real vent-man, but his name is not Kelly and he does not block traffic or shout at passersby.

33. That is, not just momentarily but in a long-term way.

34. Can there be people who are deviant *and* irrational but not deviant *because* they are irrational? No, since irrationality is itself a form of deviance. So our distinction between those who are deviant because they are irrational and those who are deviant but not irrational is exhaustive.

35. By "irrational deviant" we shall mean a person who is deviant because he is irrational.

36. See Kittrie, *The Right to be Different,* Chapter 9 for a defense of a similar position. Kittrie, however, does not allow interference if you are only a danger to yourself.
37. See Kittrie, *The Right to be Different.*
38. See McClean and DeFries, *Introduction to Behavioral Genetics* (San Francisco: W. H. Freeman, 1973), Chap. 11.

BIBLIOGRAPHY

Beauchamp, Tom L. "Paternalism and Bio-Behavioral Control." *The Monist,* Vol. 60, No. 1 (January 1977).

Beauchamp, Tom L. and Walters, LeRoy (eds.). *Contemporary Issues in Bioethics.* Belmont, Calif.: Dickenson, 1978. Chap. 11.

Kittrie, Nicholas. *The Right to be Different.* Baltimore, Md.: The Johns Hopkins Press, 1971.

Valenstein, Elliot S. *Brain Control.* New York: Wiley, 1973.

FIVE

The Right to Health Care and Its Implications

While social reformers tell us that "health is a right," the realization of that "right" is always less than complete because some of the resources that could be used for health are allocated to other purposes. . . . No country is as healthy as it could be; no country does as much for the sick as it is technically capable of doing.[1]

What the "social reformers" tell us is true—or almost true. There is no right to health, but there is—as we will argue later—a right to health care. But it is also true that "no country does as much for the sick as it is technically capable of doing" since resources that could be used for health care are in fact used for other purposes—such as justice, beauty, comfort, and education. As we will see, the need to use resources for many other goals besides health is one of the main reasons why the practical implications of the right to health care are unclear. Another is that people—trained health-care professionals—are one of the essential "resources" needed for health care, and this resource cannot be arbitrarily "allocated" where it is needed for the simple reason that people have rights which we must take into account.

So, exactly what is implied by the right to health care? To answer this question, we will focus on three socioeconomic problems connected with health and health care. The first is the problem of determining the level of health. Consider, for example, that in the United States the death rate for males in the 45 to 54 age group is about double the rate in Sweden.[2] Is this a sign of an unacceptable level of health in our society? Other things being equal, it would certainly be good to reduce the death rate in this age group. But is the present death rate acceptable—given that other things are not equal, given that we want to use our limited resources for other goals besides health? What does the right to health care imply about this situation? We will consider these issues in section 3.

The second problem is the delivery of health care. Our current system of health-care delivery creates inequalities in access to health care. Some—relatively few—easily obtain the health care they need or want while others—for a variety of reasons—have difficulty obtaining adequate health care. Do such inequalities violate the right to health care? And if they do, what should be done about it? Are the violations justified or unjustified? Section 4 will consider these issues.

Finally, there is the problem of high costs. Adequate health care is expensive and its cost is increasing. What does the right to health care imply about this situation? Does it mean that the government should ensure that each person can obtain a certain minimum level of health care no matter what his ability to pay? Section 5 focuses on these questions.

These three socioeconomic issues are part of the much broader issue of what the structure of society should be. As we said in Chapter 1, we live in a complex network of social and political relations and dependencies—a network in which each of us traces out his or her unique personal history. The question is how this network should be organized. The issue of health care is just one aspect of this question, which it will be helpful to keep in mind at points in our discussion. However, we will first explain why there is a right to health care.

1. Why is there a right to health care?

Let us recall how we earlier defined health. Roughly, we said that—in the most important sense—health is a certain state of mental and physical functioning which is conducive to self-realization.[3] Health care, then, should be understood as an attempt to restore or maintain such a state. *So, if you interfere with a person's health care, you interfere with his pursuit of self-realization;* and this means that you would be interfering with his right to self-determination—with his right to pursue those plans and projects he believes will lead to self-realization. In fact, the right to health care can be regarded as a special case of the right to self-determination, and in the section on theoretical foundations we will show in detail how to derive the right to health care from the right to self-determination.

Consider what it means to say there is a right to health care. Given our definition of what a right is, to say there is a right to health care is to say there is a reason (of a certain special sort) why others should not interfere with our health care.[4] Since the right to health care exists, such a reason against interference exists. But—in practice—what counts as interference? And when is interference justified? These are the two basic questions we must answer in considering the practical implications of the right to health care. We can illustrate these questions by considering some facts and examples of the issues mentioned earlier: determining the level of health, the delivery of health care, and the high cost of health care.

2. Facts and examples

Determining the level of health.   When polio vaccine became readily available in the fifties, the government began a massive vaccination program which proved successful in virtually eliminating polio. This campaign against polio was generally well received by the public, which must have perceived the number of polio victims as indicating an unacceptable level of health in the population. We currently have the same attitude toward cancer and heart disease. At least we are investing a great deal of time and money in such research, and it is difficult to see why we would do so if we did not perceive the number of people afflicted with cancer or heart disease as indicating an unacceptable level of health.

On the other hand, there are certain widespread types of illness that we are willing to tolerate—the common cold and the less severe forms of influenza, for example. Our lives would be much pleasanter if we had effective cures for colds and the flu, but apparently we do not regard it as worthwhile to invest much time and money in research aimed at finding such cures. So, even though colds and the flu afflict us all, we must not regard that as indicating an unacceptable level of health.

How do we determine what counts as an acceptable level of health? And once it has been determined that the level of health is unacceptable in some way, what should be done about it? Are there situations in which doing nothing about an unacceptable level of health would count as interfering with health care—and so count as a violation of the right to health care? These questions arise because the structure of society affects our individual health. The polio example illustrates this point well. Government action improved the health of many individuals by virtually eliminating polio. Would it have been a violation of the right to health care to have the capacity to virtually eliminate polio but not do so? And if it would have been, are we now violating the right to health care by not developing and using effective treatments for the flu and the common cold (if such treatments can be found)?

On what grounds are such decisions to be made? It is of some practical importance to determine what these grounds are, as decisions concerning the level of health may involve substantial risks—known or unknown. For example, between 1955 and 1961 from ten to thirty million American children were given polio shots which contained a live, possibly tumor-producing virus.[5] This was not known at the time, but in 1960 the virus was found in the kidneys of the monkeys used in the production of the polio vaccine. Fortunately, the virus has—so far as can be determined—caused no ill effects yet. If we are going to run such risks as this, we should have a good idea of the grounds on which a decision about the level of health should be made.

Health-care delivery. There are inequalities in our current system of health-care delivery. The most obvious inequality is geographical distribution. Doctors tend to concentrate in urban or suburban areas largely because there are more cultural, professional, and recreational opportunities in cities. As a consequence, people living in rural areas may have difficulty obtaining adequate health care. Now, if we allow such an unequal geographical distribution of doctors, are we interfering with the health care of people who live in rural areas—and hence violating their right to health care?

The problem of the geographical distribution of numbers of doctors is often noted, but there is also a related problem which is less often mentioned—namely, the uneven geographical distribution of the quality of health care. The fact is that the highest quality health care is found in urban and suburban areas. One reason is that there are more doctors in these areas, and so there is a greater chance of finding a knowledgeable and skillful physician. Also, the most knowledgeable doctors and the most advanced equipment tend to be found in hospitals affiliated with medical schools,[6] and such hospitals are generally found in cities. So, better health care is available in cities than in rural areas. Now, if we allow this unequal distribution of quality, do we violate the right to health care by interfering with the health care of people in rural areas? We know the inequality is there. If we do nothing about it, should we count that as interfering with health care? And if it does, is the interference justified or not?

These questions do not arise only for rural areas. Even in cities health care is unevenly distributed in both quantity and quality. High-quality health care means access to an excellent physician who is not only knowledgeable about, but also concerned about, our individual health problems and health history. In addition, access to such care should be easy and reliable. Unfortunately, relatively few people get easy and reliable access to excellent, individualistic care. There are three reasons for this.

First, there are social and economic barriers. People from the lower socioeconomic classes are often barred from obtaining health care because it costs far more than they can afford or because they are discriminated against on racial grounds.[7]

Second, there just are not that many physicians who provide first-rate, individualistic care. In recent years doctors have become highly specialized, and the number of general practitioners—now often called primary-care physicians—has declined. So, increasingly, we end up seeing Dr. A for a problem in which he specializes, Dr. B for another problem which fits his specialty, Dr. C for yet another problem, and so on. It is more difficult than it used to be to find a single doctor who will oversee the entire course of our medical care and who will know its entire history and be concerned with its overall quality.

Third, many people have difficulty obtaining individualistic health care because they do not interact effectively with their doctor. Effective interaction requires some knowledge of what a doctor can and cannot do and some knowledge about health and illness. Unfortunately, this sort of knowledge is not widespread.

It is clear, then, that there are inequalities in the distribution of health care in both quantity and quality. What does the right to health care imply about such inequalities? If we knowingly allow them to exist, are we interfering with health care and consequently violating the right to health care? Could such violations be justified?

The problem of high costs. Consider these facts:

> In 1973 Americans spent an average of $450 per person for health care and related activities such as medical education and research. This was almost 8 percent of the GNP (the gross national product is the value of all goods and services produced in the nation). Twenty years before, health care represented only 4.5 percent of the nation's output, and even as recently as 1962 health expenditures rose at the rate of 10 percent annually while the rest of the economy (as reflected in the GNP) was growing at only 6 to 7 percent.[8]

The point is that the amount of money spent on health care increased significantly between the fifties and the seventies, and the trend still continues.[9] We will not analyze why there is such a trend; instead, we will assume that it is, in part at least, an unavoidable and justifiable result of various economic and social factors.[10] For example, one reason that we pay more for health care is that there is more health care to buy. We can do much more to maintain and restore health than we were able to do in the past, but such medical skills and medical technology are costly to employ.

Our basic question will be: Given that we will be spending increasing amounts on health care, who should pay? If a person cannot afford health care that he needs, should we regard this as interfering with his health care and hence as a violation of his right to health care? In general, does the right to health care imply that the government should ensure that each person can obtain a certain minimum level of health care regardless of his ability to pay?

Now that we have surveyed the practical issues raised by the right to health care, let us turn to the detailed examination of each of the three socioeconomic problems.

3. Determining the level of health

The first point in the level-of-health issue is this: The overall structure of society affects our individual health. For example, as we already noted, the death rate in the United States for males in the 45 to 54 age group is about double what it is in Sweden. The structure of American society—with its habits of diet and exercise and its typical stresses and tensions—no doubt plays a part in creating this difference. Here is another example. Between 1900 and 1930 the death rate of infants declined very strikingly in the United States because of a sharp reduction in deaths from the pneumonia-diarrhea complex. This complex generally appears among infants living in unsanitary conditions as a result of which they contract an internal infection, leading to diarrhea, then pneumonia. The most likely cause of this sharp drop in the infant death rate was changes in the structure of social organization. a rising standard of living combined with better education and a drop in the birth rate.[11]

Clearly, then, the structure of society affects individual health. To get a general picture of how this happens, imagine the complex network of social and political relations which constitutes the structure of society. This web of sociopolitical interconnections is continually changing. Each of us changes it slightly as we trace out the unique pattern of our own life. And the actions of powerful private or governmental groups may change it significantly—either quickly and dramatically or slowly over a period of time. Now, some of these changes involve compromises about how resources—such as time, energy, money, and people—are to be used. We make such compromises because we live in a world where there are too few resources to achieve all we want to achieve. In particular, we do not do all we could to promote health and improve health care because that would cost too much in terms of resources. We have other goals we want to use those resources for—goals like education and comfort.

Now, the compromises society makes about how to use its resources affect the individuals in it, and there are two sorts of compromises which will affect our individual health. On the one hand, there are compromises between health and other nonhealth goals, and on the other hand, there are compromises among various health-related goals; for once we have decided how much to invest in health as opposed to other nonhealth goals, we still have to decide how to distribute the resources allocated to health in general. For example, we have to decide how much to invest in cancer research and how much in research on heart disease. These two sorts of compromise play an important role in determining the level of health in society.

The question on which we want to focus is: How are such compromises to be made? Now, we continually do make compromises in the area of health and health care—compromises with serious consequences for certain people. For example, we do not invest as much time, energy, labor, and money in developing treatments for rare diseases as we do in developing treatments for more common ones, even though some people will suffer and die as a result. And it is not that we lack the needed resources. We have them, but we use them for other goals even though that means it is certain that some people will suffer and die as a result of our compromise.

Even so, such compromises make good sense. To see the rationale behind compromises between health and other nonhealth goals, consider the point of being healthy, which is to be in a state conducive to self-realization. Now, given that our reason for wanting to be healthy is that it is conducive to self-realization, it does not make sense to invest all of our resources in health and health care for the simple reason that health is not the only factor conducive to self-realization. In addition to health, the pursuit of self-realization requires power to manipulate our environment, power to get what we want; so, some resources should be invested in gaining and maintaining such power. And for most of us, justice, beauty, comfort, and education are necessary to our pursuit of self-realization.

Essentially the same argument shows that we should make compromises among health-related goals. Given that we want to promote health in order to promote self-realization, we do not want to invest all of our resources in cancer research. There are many other diseases that afflict us and affect our ability to pursue self-realization, so we should invest some of our resources in treating those diseases as well.

We can see it makes sense that society should make compromises between health and other goals and also among health-related goals. And with this point we have returned to our basic question: How are such compromises to be made? If it were just a matter of one person deciding how to use his own resources independently of everyone else, the rule he should follow would be to make those compromises which maximize his self-realization since each person has good reason to try to maximize his own self-realization.[12] But what rule should we follow in making compromises for society as a whole? The answer is, of course, that we should maximize self-realization in general. But there is a problem with putting this idea into practice: namely, interpersonal conflict. A compromise which promotes your self-realization may not promote mine because of our individual differences—both physical and psychological.

The psychological differences are particularly important here. As the psychoanalyst Carl Jung points out:

> A man must have a very clouded vision, or view human society from a very misty distance, to cherish the notion that the uniform regulation of life would automatically ensure a uniform distribution of happiness. He must be pretty far gone in delusion if he imagines that equality of income, or equal opportunities for all, would have about the same value for everyone. But if he were a legislator, what would he do about all those people whose greatest opportunities lie not without but within? If he were just, he would have to give at least twice as much money to the one man as to the other, since to the one it means so much and to the other little. No social legislation will be able to overcome the psychological differences between men, this most necessary factor for generating the vital energy of a human society.[13]

Psychological differences cause great difficulties in trying to maximize self-realization for an entire society. In particular, it is difficult to see how any compromise between health and other goals can be fair to all since individual psychological differences ensure that any compromise will favor some people over others. For example, suppose that appreciating great art is far more important to your self-realization than finding a way to diagnose hemophilia in a fetus.[14] and suppose that I feel just the opposite. Then, if we invest more in art than the diagnosis of hemophilia, you are favored—while the opposite would favor me.

Of course, we might invest exactly the same amounts. We might, but this option is usually not feasible since dividing our resources evenly over all our goals often does not result in giving enough to any goal to have a chance of achieving it. For example, suppose that to have a genuine chance of finding a diagnosis for hemophilia in fetuses we need to invest a great deal of time, energy, labor, money—so much that it would be impossible to invest an equal amount in art. In such a case, an equal division of resources between these two goals would be pointless since the resources invested in hemophilia diagnosis would just be wasted.

The question of how to make compromises in the area of health and health care is clearly a problematic one. It would be a serious mistake to try to solve this problem by ignoring or attempting to minimize individual psychological differences. Enforced uniformity is not an acceptable solution. Not only would enforced uniformity violate people's rights, it would also tend to destroy those psychological differences which are—as Jung points out—essential to a vital social organization. *An acceptable solution must respect individual differences. Also, an acceptable solution should maximize the self-realization of the individuals who compose society.* The two guidelines we offer are a solution that meets these two criteria of acceptability.

These guidelines are not intended as a complete set of rules for making decisions about resources and health, but rather as a definition of the moral framework in which such decisions are to be made. A more complete answer would at least have to incorporate ideas and models from economics since that science has developed detailed approaches to the problem of reconciling conflicting individual interests. As the economist Victor Fuchs says in his book, *Who Shall Live?:*

> The major problems of health and medical care ... are high cost, poor access, and inadequate health levels. In order to attack them intelligently, we must recognize the scarcity of resources and the need to allocate them as efficiently as possible. We must recognize that we can't have everything. In short, we need to adopt an economic point of view.[15]

But Fuchs also points out that a consideration of the choices we face

> reveals some of the limits of economics in dealing with the most fundamental questions of health and medical care. The questions are ultimately ones of value: What value do we put on saving a life? on reducing pain? on relieving anxiety? How do these values change when the life at stake is a relative's? a neighbor's? a stranger's?[16]

Our concern here is with the moral side of the issue. So, let us turn to the guidelines.

The first guideline is simply this: *Maximize self-realization for society as a whole.* Now, there are two ways to do this. We can maximize the quality or quantity. We can maximize the quality of a person's self-realization by ensuring that he can realize those aspects of his ideal self-image he most desires to realize. The measure of quality is the strength of the individual person's desire. We can maximize the quantity of self-realization by promoting the self-realization of as many people as possible. Ideally, we would maximize both quantity and quality by ensuring that each person (quantity) maximized the quality of his self-realization. This is impossible to do, however, for two reasons. First, the various plans and projects of people conflict. (Recall the conflict between a doctor, who wants to save lives, and a Jehovah's Witness, who refuses a blood transfusion on religious grounds.) Second, even if there were no conflict, we do not have sufficient resources to allow people to carry out their plans and projects fully. For these two reasons, maximizing self-realization for society as a whole is always a matter of balancing quality against quantity. The second guideline is intended to define the moral boundaries within which such balancing should take place.

The second guideline is this: *No compromise between health and other goals should ever unjustifiably violate any right—in particular the right to health care.* Given that a right like the right to health care exists, it should, of course, never be unjustifiably violated. The idea behind this guideline is to ensure that there is a certain equality or fairness in the compromise since each person's rights must be respected. Suppose, for example, that society were organized in such a way that high-quality health care was available to the relatively few people who were economically well-off. Suppose also that, because of the resources invested in providing such high-quality care, a large group of poorer people have great difficulty in obtaining even adequate health care, let alone high-quality care. Such an arrangement sacrifices quantity to quality by promoting the self-realization of a few at the expense of many. Now, it is this sort of arrangement that the second guideline rules out since—as we will argue in the next section—the arrangement unjustifiably violates the right to health care.

The second guideline does not mean that everyone should be treated the same. Consider that to violate the right to health care is to interfere with a person's health care. But—because of individual differences— what interferes with your health care may not interfere with mine. Respecting the right to health care not only allows for individual differences, it actually demands that we recognize and deal with them. So, respecting the right to health care is a safeguard against uniformity and standardization.

4. The delivery of health care

We saw in section 2 that health care is unevenly distributed in both quantity and quality. Do these inequalities violate the right to health care? They certainly do. To violate the right to health care is to interfere with a person's attempt to obtain health care. If society is organized in a way that makes it difficult or impossible to obtain the health care we want or need, that organization of society violates our right to health care. Now, the facts and examples we discussed in section 2 show that our society is indeed organized in ways that make it difficult or impossible for many people to obtain the health care they want or need. Therefore, the structure of our society violates the right to health care.

This is hardly a surprising fact since even the briefest reflection reveals striking inequalities in our society. Contrast the luxury of upper Park Avenue in New York City with the lead-poisoned, rat-bitten children of Harlem. Or consider that in Philadelphia one single street— South Street—divides one of the city's richest sections from one of its poorest. Or contrast the ghettos of San Francisco and Los Angeles with the opulent areas of those cities. Our large cities are perfect images of inequality. And these inequalities violate rights—in particular, the right to health care.

The crucial question is whether these violations are justified. This is the essential issue since the rights of individuals will always be violated to some extent by any form of social organization. Now, since violations of rights are unavoidable, it is essential to be able to tell when a violation is justified and when it is not. So, how do we tell? Most of us find something unfair and objectionable about the inequalities we have noted in the social organization of the United States. As Victor Fuchs writes in *Who Shall Live?*:

> My own view is that we must quickly come to grips with the tremendous inequality in our nation. Imagine how critical we would be of a family which permitted some members to live in great luxury while other members lacked a minimum of basic goods and services? At the community level this is precisely the condition we tolerate.[17]

The answer to Fuch's question is, of course, that most of us would be extremely critical of such a family—and many of us are in fact critical of society in just this way because we think that society's inequalities unjustifiably violate people's rights.

There is a reason behind this critical reaction; namely, we can imagine a different social structure which would be socially preferable. This social structure would not only do at least as well as the current structure in maximizing the self-realization of society as a whole, but it would also be fairer—it would violate the rights of fewer people or violate them to a lesser degree. The basis of our criticism of the family would be essentially the same; we can see a different way in which to organize the family—a fairer way which would be equally good at maximizing self-realization. Basically, we would insist on a more even distribution of goods and services in the family. Of course, this would decrease the quality of self-realization of those who benefit from the current arrangement, but this decrease would be counterbalanced by the increase in the quality of self-realization of those benefited by the change. Recall here that we can maximize self-realization in two ways—by either quality or quantity. In the family case the increase in quantity compensates for the decreases in quality. The same happens in society as a whole. (We will not discuss the problem of balancing quality against quantity.)

Focusing on the family illustrates another important point. We would not criticize the family as unfair if the way in which it was organized was—for some good reason—the only way in which it could be organized. In such a case the family members would be doing as well as they could do; it would be unfortunate that they could not do better, but we would have to regard the violation of rights involved as justified. Likewise, we would not regard the structure of social organization as unjustifiably violating rights if that form of organization were the only feasible one. For the violations to be unjustified, the different, socially preferable organization has to be a feasible alternative; that is, it has to be possible to transform the present social structure into the different, socially preferable structure without paying too high a price in terms of the violation of rights and the frustration of desires. We can illustrate the idea of paying too high a price with the following example. Suppose someone proposed we immediately remodel our health-care system along the lines of a socialist system such as Sweden's. And suppose—for the sake of argument—that this change would ultimately result in a socially preferable structure. Even so, forcing this change immediately on our society is objectionable since it would so drastically violate the rights and frustrate the desires of health-care professionals and their patients.

To summarize: A right is unjustifiably violated by the structure of social organization if there is a socially preferable structure which is a feasible alternative.[18] The right to health care is justifiably violated by the structure of our society provided there is a socially preferable structure (involving health care) which is a feasible alternative to our present system of health care. Is there such a way to reorganize our society? If there is, our society unjustifiably violates the right to health care. The best way to argue that a socially preferable and feasible alternative exists in the area of health is to describe it in detail. Now, any description of this sort would have to include a complicated consideration of economic and sociological factors which are not our concern here. I do want to claim, however, that there is a socially preferable organization of the health care system which is a feasible alternative to our present system.

We can illustrate this claim by examining one aspect of our current health-care system and explaining how and why that aspect should be changed. The fact is that many industries, such as insurance companies, drug companies, and nursing homes, profit from illness. In such cases, the motive to make a profit exists side by side with the motive to provide health care. These two motives need not conflict, but the clear fact of the matter is that they often do. And health care suffers as a result, for what often happens is that the cause of profit making is served at the expense of providing adequate health care.

The drug industry is a good example. The rate of profit from drugs is very high—approximately sixty cents of every dollar.[19] Fuchs comments on this situation in *Who Shall Live?*:

> There can be little doubt that drug prices could be reduced substantially if sharp cuts were made in advertising, research expenditures, and profits. Whether this would be desirable or not is another matter. It is naive to assume that the public interest always lies in the direction of lower prices. If lowering prices were to inhibit the development of useful new drugs, for instance, the public interest might be poorly served.
>
> High profits have probably helped fuel the rapid expansion of the drug industry in the past. If there is less need for expansion now, profits could and probably should be lower. The charge that expenditures for drug marketing are excessive seems well supported, but these expenditures are likely to continue as long as they pay off for the manufacturers.[20]

If profits were lower—as they should be—drug prices could be lower. This would contribute to holding down the cost of health care, and that would allow more people to obtain adequate care while still allowing drug manufacturers a reasonable profit. So, reorganizing the health-care system so that drug company profits were lowered would both promote self-realization and be fairer—that is, the right to health care would be violated less often and to a lesser degree.[21] This means that such a reorganization would be socially preferable since it does at least as good a job of maximizing self-realization while at the same time being fairer.

But is the reorganization a feasible alternative to our present system? That is, can we transform our present system into one in which drug company profits are lower without paying too high a cost in the violations of people's rights and the frustration of their desires? I think the answer is *yes*, but showing this requires a detailed examination of economic and sociological facts. The basic problem is that drug profits can probably be adequately controlled only by some form of government intervention and regulation (although this could be debated).[22]

To argue that the reorganization we suggest is a feasible alternative we would have to specify the form of regulation to be used, and we would have to show that imposing this form of regulation did not violate too many rights or frustrate too many desires. I think this could be shown for a suitable system of regulation, but we will not argue the point here.

The drug manufacturer example was only intended to illustrate the claim that there is a socially preferable organization of the health-care system which is a feasible alternative to our present system. There are many factors which would have to be considered in a full treatment of this issue—for example, the unequal distribution of health care in both quantity and quality. What, if anything, should be done about unequal distribution? While our aim has been to develop a moral framework within which such questions can be raised and answered, we should emphasize the need for a detailed and careful consideration of economic and sociological factors in answering them. Proposals about what is socially preferable and about what constitutes a feasible alternative must be based on an adequate examination of the facts. We should have little patience for proposals about what is just or fair in society if these proposals are blind to the realities of our social life.

5. The problem of high costs

One of the realities of our social life is the rapidly increasing cost of health care, and as we pointed out in section 2, this trend is—at least in part—an inevitable and justifiable result of various sociological and economic factors. The question we asked was: Given that the cost of health care will continue to increase, who should pay for it? The answer, I think, must be that the government will have to bear an increasing responsibility for ensuring that people can obtain a certain minimum level of health care no matter what their ability to pay. Now, in fact, the government has already taken on this responsibility through a variety of programs—for example, Medicare. Indeed, we are currently involved in a transformation of our health-care system. Years ago paying for health care was primarily the responsibility of an individual or his family. Gradually, that system has changed into one in which the government plays a large role—directly or indirectly—in financing the health care of a significant portion of the population. A justification of this developing system would have to compare it to other possible systems to see which one best maximized self-realization and also to see which one was fairer—to see which system violated fewer rights or violated them to a lesser degree. To justify the developing system we would have to argue that it represented the best compromise open to us between the two goals of maximizing self-realization and being fair.

I think we could argue convincingly that some form or other of government support for health care does represent the best compromise open to us. But we will not argue this point; we will just assume it is true. Instead, we will turn our attention to a problem which inevitably arises with government financing of health care—the problem of bureaucracy.

Any form of government financing of health care will involve the formation of a bureaucracy; and as Waitzkin and Waterman, two sociologists concerned with health care, point out:

> The dehumanizing and alienating manifestations of bureaucracy have made themselves felt in many socialist countries which have tried to establish effective health-care systems. . . . As a result patients often face cumbersome procedures which inhibit their ability to obtain the health care that they seek.[23]

Our concern here will not be with solving the problems of bureaucracy[24] but with understanding why certain aspects of bureaucracy are objectionable. To guard against danger it is best to be able to recognize it.

As Waitzkin and Waterman note, the most morally objectionable feature of bureaucracy is that it is "dehumanizing and alienating." An individual is not treated as an individual but as a cog in a vast operation in which individual differences and individual peculiarities and needs are sacrificed in the name of overall efficiency. In the case of health care this can happen to health-care professionals as well as to patients. While it is certainly true that, confronted with an elaborate bureaucracy, "patients often face cumbersome procedures which inhibit their ability to obtain the health care which they seek," it is also true that bureaucracy can severely restrict the freedom of action of doctors and other health-care professionals. I do not see any justification for creating a bureaucracy which dictates procedures and treatments and thereby robs health-care professionals of the freedom to use their judgment. I also see no justification for a bureaucracy which does not allow health-care professionals the same freedom of choice about where to live, when to work, and so on as other professional people are allowed.

The basic problem is that of balancing individual freedom against the collective demands of society. The demands of society force themselves on us when we see the misery, pain, and suffering which exist, in part, because of the inequalities of our social organization. If we are to respect rights—such as the right to health care—we should do what we can to eliminate these inequalities. But eliminating inequalities often means restricting individual freedom—in the case of health care by the creation of a complicated bureaucracy.

The irony of the situation is that to protect the right to health care we have to create a bureaucracy which threatens individuality. But respecting the right to health care also demands that we take account of individual differences and needs. An acceptable solution to the problem of high costs must protect individual freedom by recognizing and allowing for individual physical and psychological differences.

6. Conclusion

It is fitting that this book should end with a plea for the importance of the individual. Our moral perspective has emphasized the importance of the individual, of his capabilities for free choice and rational judgment, and so it seems appropriate to repeat the quote from Carl Jung with which we concluded the first chapter:

In the face of huge numbers every thought of individuality pales, for statistics obliterate everything unique. Contemplating such overwhelming might and misery, the individual is embarrassed to exist at all. Yet the real carrier of life is the individual. He alone feels happiness, he alone has virtue and responsibility and any ethics whatever. The masses and the state have nothing of the kind.

THEORETICAL FOUNDATIONS

We need to see why there is a right to health care, and to do that we should recall the concept of health we developed in Chapter 2. We defined the basic concept of health as—roughly—a state of physical and mental functioning which is conducive to self-realization. It is in this sense of *health* that a person has a right to health care. By our definition of what a right is, this right exists if and only if (1) there is a reason why others should not interfere with your health care, and (2) each person has this reason simply by virtue of being a person.

Do (1) and (2) hold? To see that (1) does, consider that when a person seeks health care, he is attempting to maintain or restore a state of physical and mental functioning which is conducive to self-realization. Now, there is a reason why we should not interfere with such attempts. This follows from the right to self-determination. To say that we have the right to self-determination is to say two things: (1') there is a reason why others should not interfere with our pursuit of those plans and projects which we believe will lead to our self-realization, and (2') each person has this reason simply by virtue of being a person.

It is (1') that makes (1) true. Or more exactly, it is (1') plus the fact that to interfere with our health care—in the sense of *health* noted above—is one way to interfere with our pursuit of self-realization. Given this fact, it follows immediately from (1') that (1) holds—there is a reason why others should not interfere with our health care. Now, does (2) hold? Does each person have this reason simply by virtue of being a person? Given (2'), the answer must be *yes*. We have derived the reason in question from (1'), and (2') tells us that each person has that reason simply by virtue of being a person. We can conclude, therefore, that there is a right to health care.

FURTHER QUESTIONS

1. What should be done about the unequal geographical distribution of health care in both quantity and quality?

2. Would our resources be better used in finding treatments for common illnesses like the flu rather than searching for cures to cancer and treatments for heart disease?

3. How—if at all—can the developing system of government-financed health care be justified?

4. Should taxes be raised to help support government-financed health care?

NOTES

1. Victor R. Fuchs, *Who Shall Live?* (New York: Basic Books, 1974), p. 17.
2. Ibid, p. 15.
3. Chapter 2, p. 61.
4. See Introduction, p. 12.
5. Reported in Michael Rogers, *Biohazard* (New York: Knopf, 1977), p. 34. The virus is SV-40.

6. *Who Shall Live?*, p. 89.
7. It is worth pointing out that economic barriers can also bar members of the middle class from obtaining health care. A prolonged illness which requires more hospitalization than a middle-class family's insurance covers can be a financial disaster. Such a family can be worse off in terms of health care than a lower-class family which is eligible for state aid.
8. *Who Shall Live?*, p. 10.
9. Howard B. Waitzkin and Barbara Waterman, *The Exploitation of Illness in Capitalist Society* (Indianapolis, Ind.: Bobbs-Merrill, 1974), pp. 8–16, contains an interesting analysis of this trend.
10. See *Who Shall Live?*, Chap. 6.
11. Ibid., p. 32.
12. See Introduction, p. 11.
13. Carl Jung, *Psychological Types* (Princeton, N.J.: Princeton University Press, 1971), p. 487.
14. There is currently no satisfactory way to test for hemophilia in a fetus in utero.
15. *Who Shall Live?*, p. 29.
16. Ibid, p. 29.
17. Ibid, p. 118.
18. This is only a sufficient condition. We will not attempt to state a necessary and sufficient condition.
19. *Who Shall Live?*, p. 121.
20. Ibid, pp. 121–122.
21. This could be debated, but we will assume it is true.
22. Various issues relevant to this point are discussed in *Who Shall Live?*
23. *The Exploitation of Illness in Capitalist Society*, pp. 109–110.
24. Ibid, contains some suggestions; see pp. 108–116.

BIBLIOGRAPHY

Freidson, Eliot. *Professional Dominance.* Chicago: Aldine, 1970.

Fuchs, Victor R. *Who Shall Live?* New York: Basic Books, 1974.

Rawls, John. *A Theory of Justice.* Cambridge, Mass.: Harvard University Press, 1971.

Waitzkin, Howard B., and Waterman, Barbara. *The Exploitation of Illness in Capitalist Society.* Indianapolis, Ind.: Bobbs-Merrill, 1974.

Index

NAME INDEX